DEVIL IN THE MILK

DEVIL IN THE MILK

Illness, health, and the politics of A1 and A2 milk

KEITH WOODFORD

Foreword by
THOMAS COWAN, MD

Chelsea Green Publishing
White River Junction, Vermont

AUTHOR'S NOTE

Where scientists play a major role in the milk devil story, and where their titles are known (either Professor or Doctor) I use those titles when first mentioning a person. I also use the given name. However, for some scientists, particularly those mentioned primarily as authors, neither title nor given name is evident from their publications. Most medical scientists will hold the degree of PhD (or its European equivalent) and have the title of Doctor. However, some scientists have different qualifications that may or may not provide the title of Doctor. I apologise to any scientist mentioned in this book without use of title who considers that a title should have been used. On occasions there may also be inconsistency in the use of given names. This can arise when scientists from non-English–speaking countries use both anglicised and non-anglicised versions. Where names are used widely within the same section, for brevity I usually repeat only the surname.

First published in 2007 by Craig Potton Publishing
98 Vickerman Street, PO Box 555, Nelson, New Zealand

Printed in the United States of America
First Chelsea Green printing, March 2009
10 9 8 7 6 5 4 3 11 12

Our Commitment to Green Publishing
Chelsea Green sees publishing as a tool for cultural change and ecological stewardship. We strive to align our book manufacturing practices with our editorial mission and to reduce the impact of our business enterprise in the environment. We print our books and catalogs on chlorine-free recycled paper, using vegetable-based inks whenever possible. This book may cost slightly more because it was printed on paper that contains recycled fiber, and we hope you'll agree that it's worth it. Chelsea Green is a member of the Green Press Initiative (www.greenpressinitiative.org), a nonprofit coalition of publishers, manufacturers, and authors working to protect the world's endangered forests and conserve natural resources. *Devil in the Milk* was printed on FSC®-certified paper supplied by Thomson-Shore that contains at least 30% postconsumer recycled fiber.

Library of Congress Cataloging-in-Publication Data
Woodford, K. B.
Devil in the milk : illness, health and politics : A1 and A2 milk / Keith Woodford.
p. cm.
"First published in 2007 by Craig Potton Publishing."
Includes bibliographical references and index.
ISBN 978-1-60358-102-8
1. Milk--Health aspects. 2. Casein--Pathophysiology. I. Title.

RA602.M54W66 2009
613.2'6--dc22

2009000817

Chelsea Green Publishing Company
Post Office Box 428
White River Junction, VT 05001
(802) 295-6300
www.chelseagreen.com

CONTENTS

FOREWORD

My career as a physician, which now spans over 25 years, has been closely linked to milk and other dairy products. That connection is thanks in part to a book I came across early in my medical training—*The Milk of Human Kindness Is not Pasteurized,* by William Campbell Douglass, MD, a true medical rebel. It turned out to be one of the most important books on medicine that I have ever read, and it helped form my views on medicine. (The book has since been republished as *The Milk Book.*)

Fueled by Dr. Douglass's insights, I quickly became an advocate for raw milk and saw a lot of positive benefits from switching people from commercial pasteurized milk and milk products to pasture-fed, raw, and cultured dairy. Already, I had long been an advocate for eating butter and other full-fat products—another stance that has been largely vindicated by current medical research as well as the catastrophe that is margarine. This phase was followed by my introduction to *Nourishing Traditions* by Sally Fallon—another passionate full-fat, raw-milk advocate—and the subsequent founding of the Weston A. Price Foundation, of which I am one of the founding board members. I then authored *The Fourfold Path to Healing,* along with Sally and Jaimen McMillan, which among other things spoke of the dangers of commercial pasteurized dairy products and the health, social, and economic benefits that would come from our country switching to properly raised cows providing full-fat, raw dairy products.

However, all this time, I had the sense that somehow I didn't have the full story. In my practice, I was continually faced with patients whose medical situation improved only once they had stopped cow's milk entirely. Butter and ghee didn't seem to cause problems, but I still saw patients whose immune systems didn't heal or who had excess congestion and its attendant problems as long as they consumed any kind of cow's milk. Something was still up.

In *Devil in the Milk*, Farm Management and Agribusiness Professor Keith Woodford delivers what seems to be a key to answering why problems persist when some patients ingest milk. As the author explains, there is a protein called beta-casein in the milk-solid part of cow's milk—but not in the fat (butter) and not in the whey. The type of beta-casein varies in cows according to their genetic makeup, but the most common types are known as A1 beta-casein and A2 beta-casein. A1Beta-casein, common in American and European cows, releases an opiate-like chemical upon digestion called BCM-7, which is the exact culprit in the myriad of symptoms I have seen all these years. These symptoms include joint and muscle pains, fatigue, digestive disturbances, and headaches. A1 beta-casein refers to the type of beta-casein that has histidine instead of proline at position 67 of the protein chain. As a result of this mutation from proline to histidine, the peptide that emerges from this amino is able to be liberated in the digestive tract of the animal or person consuming the milk. To simplify this, the cows themselves are either called A1 or A2 cows, depending on which beta-casein variant they have.

Devil in the Milk is a monumental study, convincingly laid out, and one that demands our immediate attention. If Woodford is correct, which I have no doubt he is, the effects of drinking milk from A1 cows is a piece of the puzzle that needs to be addressed. Dairy products, when properly produced and treated, have nourished generations of the healthiest humans who ever lived. If we can use this book to convert our cows to A2 cows, then use the principles of properly fed, properly prepared dairy, we will do much to reduce the disease burden in our country and find our way to the robust health that is our birthright. I encourage everyone to read this book and see for themselves.

Thomas Cowan, MD

PREFACE TO THE NORTH AMERICAN EDITION

When I wrote the first edition of this book, I wrote for a New Zealand and Australian audience. This was because much of the early work on A1 beta-casein and its health effects took place in New Zealand and to a lesser extent Australia. Also, these are my 'home audiences'. But the issue of A1 beta-casein and its health effects is a matter of huge importance throughout much of the world, particularly those countries that have 'black and white' cows of European origin. The USA, Canada, Britain, and much of Scandinavia come into this category.

Currently, very few people in North America know anything about A1 beta-casein, or the alternative milk that is free of A1 beta-casein, and which is known as A2 milk. Unlike Australia and New Zealand, A2 milk is not available in North American supermarkets. However, the main industry players in North America do have a large file on the topic and are watching closely.

International trade in dairy products is dominated by my home country, New Zealand. This includes large quantities of casein that are exported to North America by our dominant milk-marketing cooperative, Fonterra. Most American readers of this book will never have previously heard of Fonterra, but, if they have ever purchased a muesli bar or similar, there is a fair chance that the material that binds it all together is casein from Fonterra. Some of the infant formula consumed in North America will also be made from milk powder that comes from Fonterra in New Zealand.

North Americans should not be concerned that some of their casein comes from New Zealand's Fonterra. In fact, New Zealand is quietly converting its herds to A2 without telling the rest of the world. What North Americans should be concerned about is that North American milk is very high in A1 beta-casein, and almost no-one is doing anything about it.

ACKNOWLEDGEMENTS

Researching and writing this book, largely at nights and weekends and over a period of some three years, has been a solitary experience. I therefore acknowledge foremost my family, and particularly my wife Annette, who has had to put up with my pre-occupation. My family has also been an important sounding board at critical times.

Dr Andrew Clarke was particularly helpful in leading me to some of the relevant literature. I admire the way that Andrew combines a commitment to the cause of A2 milk with a stance of scientific caution, and a steadfast belief that arguments must be evidence-based.

Mike Bradstock worked closely with me as editor. His own scientific background and questioning attitude were invaluable. Mike also made a major stylistic contribution.

Julian Bateson and Don Cameron both read early drafts and helped provide me with confidence that a complex story did indeed hang together.

Robbie Burton and his team at Craig Potton Publishing have been enthusiastic and professional. It takes a brave publisher to commit to a book such as this. I like the commitment at CPP to publishing books which they believe are important.

Of course this book could never have been written without some outstanding work by many scientists who made the discoveries on which this book is based. Some of them I have met and corresponded with; others I know only by the scientific evidence that they have produced.

One always hopes that a book such as this is free of scientific error. But science is seldom free of error. Indeed the way that scientific knowledge progresses is by refutation of theories that conventional wisdom says are correct. If there are errors in this book then they are my responsibility.

PROLOGUE

This book is about the effects on human health of a tiny protein fragment called beta-casomorphin-7, or BCM7 for short.

BCM7 is unquestionably a powerful opioid and hence a narcotic. It is also an oxidant. It is formed by digestion of a particular type of milk protein produced by some cows. This milk protein is called A1 beta-casein.

The BCM7 that is released from A1 beta-casein has been implicated in many illnesses, including heart disease, Type 1 diabetes and autism. More recently it has been linked to delayed development in genetically susceptible babies that are fed infant formula. And there is increasing evidence that it is associated with milk intolerance and an additional range of auto-immune diseases. Metaphorically, it is 'the devil in the milk'.

The 'milk devil' story is built upon more than a hundred scientific papers published in international journals, and also upon documents from milk-marketing companies. It is a story that has never been brought together before.

There is strong evidence that the milk devil is only produced from the milk of cows that are of European origin, and then only from some of these cows. Asian and African breeds of cows are free of it (unless they have some hidden European ancestry). So are goats. And so, with a very minor but fascinating qualification, is human milk.

No-one can tell by looking at a cow whether or not she is a source of the milk devil. However, genetic testing is possible, and it is also possible to test the milk. Farmers can breed cows that are free of the problematic protein by using appropriately tested bulls and semen.

Anyone who buys ordinary milk at the supermarket can be sure that it will contain milk from many cows and therefore there will be lots of A1 beta-casein in it. However, the level varies between countries, and even between regions. Some countries such as Australia, New Zealand, Finland, the United States and Britain have high levels of this protein. Others, such as Iceland, France and the island of Guernsey, have much lower levels.

We don't have to stop drinking cows' milk to avoid this devil. But we do have to drink milk from cows that have been tested and found to be free of what is called the A1 variant (or 'allele') of the beta-casein gene. Milk that is free of A1 beta-casein is known as A2 milk. All milk used to be A2 milk until a natural mutation affected some European cows a long time ago.

A2 milk is available in all major Australian supermarkets. It is also available in a limited number of stores in New Zealand. During 2008 it was available in the USA through the Hy-Vee supermarket chain in seven Midwestern states, but the marketing launch was not successful and it was then withdrawn. A relaunch seems likely in 2011 or 2012. This illustrates the complexity of marketing a new product for which the messages are complex, and in competition with mainstream milk. Similarly, in other developed countries A2 milk is not currently available in the supermarkets, although in some Asian countries it is available as the generic form of milk from indigenous cows. The reasons why A2 milk continues to have a low market profile in most parts of the world is itself a major part of the story.

Throughout this book I often refer to A1 milk. This is essentially a shorthand term for milk that contains some A1 beta-casein, the source of the milk devil.

The story of A1 versus A2 milk may sound stranger than fiction. Indeed, it is an amazing story. It is a story of how science works and doesn't work. It is also a story of how the forces of big business and the so-called 'health industry' work, and of how wishful thinking can get in the way of truth.

The first edition of *Devil in the Milk* was published in 2007. An American edition was first published in 2009. In this updated American edition, events are updated through to October 2010 in a revised postscript.

INTRODUCTION

I am often asked why I have such an interest in A2 milk, and why I have taken to speaking in public about the issue. It is a valid question, because we live in a world where people are often driven by hidden motives. There is also another question, sometimes left unstated, as to whether I have the competency to talk about such matters.

I prefer to address these issues head-on, and so will explain something of my own background. But in the final analysis, my arguments and perspectives should stand or fall on the quality of the evidence. What I try to do is to provide a balanced perspective of that evidence, including the arguments of those who do not believe in what is sometimes called 'the A2 hypothesis'.

My personal intention has been to read everything in the scientific literature that seems relevant to the issue, and to treat all evidence with scepticism. This is not an easy task. For a start, the relevant literature spans research into diabetes, heart disease, autism and schizophrenia. It also includes biochemistry, pharmacology and genetics (human and bovine). Scientific journals in each of these fields have their own specialist language. Making judgements about the A2 hypothesis also requires an understanding of biometrics (the testing and interpretation of biological data) and an understanding of research processes and philosophies.

It has been interesting for me to find that there are very few people who have read widely across the literature in relation to A1 and A2 milk. This deficiency is at least in part because we live in a reductionist world where specialisation requires people to put boundaries around issues. Back in the days of Darwin, scientists from different disciplines read each other's work, but today in general that no longer occurs.

My early formal training was a four-year degree in agricultural science from Lincoln College, at that time part of Canterbury University, in New Zealand. Subsequently I studied for a Master of Agricultural Science, specialising in agricultural systems and management. Much later I undertook a PhD degree at University of Queensland in Australia, focusing on the bio-economics of industry development. Much of my professional life has been spent in and around universities. I have lived mainly in New Zealand and Australia, but also worked on development projects in more than 20 Asian and Pacific countries such as Papua New Guinea, Fiji, Cambodia and Vietnam. I have also squeezed in quite a lot of mountaineering, particularly but not exclusively in my younger days, and this has taken me around the world including Antarctica, South America and the Himalayas.

Currently I am Professor of Farm Management and Agribusiness within the Division of Agriculture and Life Sciences at Lincoln University in New Zealand. My professional interests relate to agriculture as a field of study that crosses the boundaries of science, economics, management and commerce. In the final analysis, agriculture is about people and the decisions they make, at least as much as it is about biology. At heart, I would characterise myself as an agriculturalist with particular interests in farming systems, farming decisions, and the linkages within the overall value chain from consumers back to the farm. These interests force me to read across the disciplines. Because the A2 milk issue crosses all of the normal disciplinary boundaries, it is exactly the sort of thing I enjoy getting my teeth into.

No-one can know everything in relation to the science of BCM7. There is always more to know. Biology and medicine are seldom simple. They are like a big jigsaw puzzle. In the case of BCM7, more and more of the pieces of that puzzle have been coming together. Occasionally a piece may get wrongly placed, and there can be disputes about these individual pieces and where they fit.

It has not been my job to construct the individual pieces of the puzzle. That has been the task of many specialist scientists. Given the range of disciplines involved, it would be impossible for any one person, or indeed a group of people, to construct more than a few individual pieces. My task has been to help bring together the available pieces of scientific information to illuminate the big picture. All of the key scientific information comes from published scientific papers. In this book I share this evidence, including both what we do and do not know, with you, the reader. It seems to me that this big picture has been getting progressively clearer, but you can draw your own conclusions.

As a professor of farm management and agribusiness I am interested in assessing risks to our agricultural industries and then working on strategies that farmers and downstream agribusinesses can use to minimise those risks. In relation to A2 milk it is not particularly difficult to convert a herd of cows so that they produce only A2 milk, but it typically takes about 10 years (roughly two generations of cows) to make the change. Therefore, if the issue of A1 versus A2 milk becomes important to a lot of consumers, farmers will have needed to start acting before the market demands that they do so. Also, during the period of transition there are marketing issues as to how a company can position both A1 and A2 milk in the marketplace. In a professional context, these are the types of issues that I have to address. I therefore find myself talking to farmers in New Zealand, Australia, the Americas and Europe about the business risks of moving to produce A2 milk when subsequent events may prove it was not necessary, versus the risks of not making the move and then finding that the marketplace demands that milk be the A2 variant.

Prior to November 2003 my knowledge about A1 and A2 milk was minimal. I was vaguely aware that there was a company called A2 Corporation and that it was claiming to have milk that was healthier than so-called 'normal' milk. This milk had recently gone on sale in both Australia and New Zealand. I was also aware that Fonterra, the major milk-processing and marketing co-operative in New Zealand, and also a major force within the Australian industry, was disputing the claims of A2 Corporation. (Fonterra is also by far the world's largest international trader of dairy products.) I had assumed that if Fonterra said the claims were not valid, then that was probably true.

My perspective changed totally as the result of a casual inquiry of a colleague. At the time I was a member of the Telford Rural Polytechnic Council, which meets regularly in its governance role. The Chair of the Council at that time was Dr Jock Allison, a well-known agricultural scientist who in 2003 won Lincoln University's Bledisloe Medal for the alumnus who had contributed the most to New Zealand agriculture.

One Friday morning in November 2003 I flew from Christchurch, where I live, to Dunedin, and then drove to Balclutha for one of our regular Council meetings. I had recently become aware that Jock had become a director of A2 Corporation. During a break in the meeting I asked him why he had got involved with such a company, given the questions as to the validity of the A2 Corporation's claims. Jock's response was to pull out some papers from his briefcase and tell me to read them.

On returning to Christchurch that night I was sufficiently intrigued to begin a computer search for more information. I ended up spending most of the weekend reading more and more about it. By the end of the weekend I was persuaded that the A2 hypothesis 'had legs'. I was convinced that it was going to become a really big issue and not going to go away in a hurry. I knew that I would have to do a lot more reading to get my mind around some very complex issues, and that there would be many twists and turns, with evidence and counter-evidence, argument and counter-argument, before the final truth would emerge.

Subsequent to this, but before I had a clear intention of writing extensively about A1 beta-casein and BCM7, some of my family, but not me personally, purchased a minor shareholding in A2 Corporation. These shares were purchased on the New Zealand Stock Exchange in the same way and at the same price that any citizen could obtain them. It could therefore be argued that I was no longer completely independent in relation to these matters. On the other hand, when I first started to tell my colleagues about the A2 hypothesis, and put forward the view that it seemed to have considerable merit, one of them told me that it would be much more convincing if I 'put my money where my mouth was'. What I have learned long ago is that it is not possible to keep everyone happy. In regard to a controversy such as A1 and A2 there will be detractors whatever stance one takes. Accordingly, in articles that I wrote thereafter, I disclosed my interest, such as it was, and left people to make their own judgements. Most publishers printed the disclosure, but others chose not to, presumably on the grounds that they deemed it of no significance.

More recently, it became apparent that some people, struggling to find flaws in the evidence I presented, were indeed going to use this share ownership issue to argue that I was not independent and was writing articles for ulterior motives. It was a distraction that I did not need. Accordingly, following family discussions, the Woodford family has sold those shares. I therefore advise that neither I nor my family have any financial interest in either A2 Corporation or any franchisee thereof. I also advise that I have undertaken no consultancies for A2 Corporation, or for any joint venture company or franchisee associated with A2 Corporation.

I make the observation that disclosure of interest, and the potential for conflict of interest, can be a very tricky issue. The reality is that most people involved with the issue of A2 milk have potential conflicts of interest. That includes all dairy farmers, the dairy marketing companies, and also the scientists who depend on industry funding. I will talk more about those issues throughout this book. What we all have to endeavour to do is to recognise and disclose our interests and act with integrity in the search for truth.

I have been fascinated by the number of inherently good people who say to me 'but we must not do anything that damages the dairy industry'. When I respond that this sounds very much like the historical attitudes within the tobacco industry they are shocked by the comparison. Integrity requires that we go wherever the path of evidence takes us.

The A2 story is complex and sorting out the wheat from the chaff has not been particularly easy.

My personal assessment of the evidence is that the issue of A1 and A2 milk is a major health issue. It is also my assessment that some people have acted, either purposefully or accidentally, in a way that has obscured the truth. It is very easy to ignore unpleasant evidence that threatens an existing stance. It is a human trait. After reading this book you can make your own judgements on these matters.

Despite being a proponent of A2 milk, I do not wish to make any suggestion regarding investment in A2 Corporation. Although I am very confident that in fifty years' time, and hopefully much sooner, we will all be drinking milk that is free of A1 beta-casein, I have no clear view whether or not A2 Corporation is a good investment. Nevertheless, I do believe that A2 Corporation is very important: without it the message about A1 beta-casein and BCM7 would probably have been buried, or at least taken a great deal longer to emerge. But it is another matter whether or not A2 Corporation can prosper from its patents and trademarks. Capitalising on intellectual property is not always easy. There are lots of pitfalls, as readers of this book will become aware.

I also want to make a statement about the freedom of speech that goes with being an academic. The considered opinions and judgements that I make in this book are entirely my own. When academics speak about an issue they are representing themselves and not the university that employs them. Speaking about issues is part of our role. As academics we do not seek permission to speak on any particular issue, and we should never imply that the stance we take is the university's position. This is quite different from the situation of scientists who work for commercial organisations or for non-university government research organisations.

It is an important distinction. My employer, Lincoln University, holds no position either for or against the putative role played by what I call the milk devil.

So why have I written this book? Some of my friends have suggested to me that from a career perspective it is not a very smart move. They may be correct. But I have now got to a stage in life where some things are more important than others. I believe the A2 story is one that needs to be told.

CHAPTER ONE

BEGINNINGS

The A2 story starts in 1993 with Professor Bob Elliott from Auckland University in New Zealand. Elliott was Professor (now Professor Emeritus) of Child Health, and as part of his work had been looking at the incidence of Type 1 diabetes among Samoan children. Type 1 diabetes is an immune-response disease where the pancreas loses its ability to produce insulin. Insulin is a natural hormone required for the transport of glucose into the cells, where the glucose provides energy. The disease usually strikes either in childhood or early adulthood, but only a small proportion of people seems to be susceptible. People with Type 1 diabetes need regular insulin injections for the rest of their life. The incidence of Type 1 diabetes has been steadily rising throughout the world and it has been a real puzzle as to why this is happening. Another puzzle is why the incidence of the disease varies greatly (as much as 300-fold) between countries.

There are two types of diabetes, Type 1 and Type 2. Type 1 usually develops in childhood or young adulthood, while Type 2 is mainly a disease of older people. Both diseases relate to an inability to metabolise glucose, and both are linked to insulin, but they are also fundamentally different. Type 1 diabetics do not produce the insulin they need because of damage to the insulin-producing cells in the pancreas. In contrast, Type 2 diabetics still produce at least some insulin but their body is 'insulin resistant'. This means that the insulin, although present, cannot do a good job of getting glucose into the cells where it is needed. The way to prevent or greatly reduce the risk of Type 2 diabetes is through exercise and weight control. In contrast, there are no generally accepted health strategies for avoiding Type 1 diabetes. Our interest in this book is with Type 1 diabetes.

Bob Elliott was aware that Samoan children living in New Zealand were very susceptible to Type 1 diabetes, whereas Samoan children living in Samoa had an extremely low incidence. The tenfold difference could be explained only by an environmental or dietary factor. Elliott suspected that at least part of the answer related to the consumption of milk, which was much lower in Samoa. But he also knew that the complete answer was unlikely to be anywhere near as simple as that.

Accordingly, some time in 1993 Elliott telephoned the New Zealand Dairy Research Institute (NZDRI) and asked to speak to someone who knew about cows and milk-protein biochemistry. Dr Jeremy Hill took the call. His advice was that it could be worth looking at the beta-casein proteins, although it would be a long shot.

Hill would have known that in cattle there are essentially two major types of beta-casein protein, known as A1 and A2. There are also some other minor variants within the A1 and A2 families, but at this stage of the story they can be ignored.

The beta-casein proteins found in cattle comprise 209 amino acids in a fixed sequence and making up a convoluted string. The difference between the A1 and A2 variants is just one of these 209 amino acids. Whereas A1 milk has the amino acid histidine at position 67, the A2 milk contains proline at the same position. Back in 1993 the significance of this minor difference was not understood, although it had been known to milk biochemists for about 25 years.

The prevalence of the A1 and A2 beta-casein protein varies from one herd of cows to another, and also between countries. However, the A1 version of the gene is found only among cattle in the western world, all of which belong to the subspecies *Bos taurus*. Asian cattle are of the subspecies *Bos indicus* and do not produce A1 beta-casein.[1] African cattle, although mainly *Bos taurus*, also do not produce A1 beta-casein. However, a qualification needs to be made in that many supposedly 'pure' Asian and African cattle contain genes that can only have come from breeding with European cattle at some time in the last few thousand years, and hence may produce some A1 beta-casein. Scientists think that a mutation occurred about 8000 years ago, such that the proline at position 67 was replaced by histidine. The genetic evidence for this mutation is very clear, although there could be an error of some thousands of years as to when it occurred.[2] This mutation has subsequently been spread widely throughout herds in the western world. However, there is considerable difference in the prevalence of the A1 gene between breeds, countries, and in some cases, provinces.

So the hypothesis that Bob Elliott set out to investigate was that the risk of getting Type 1 diabetes would depend on the amount of milk that was drunk and the proportion of A1 protein in that milk. The key risk factor would be the volume of milk multiplied by its A1 content.

Undertaking human trials to investigate such issues is very difficult. The subjects of the trial would need to be identified as babies and then put on either A1 or A2 formula milk once breastfeeding ceased. The trials would probably need to go on for many years, and the children prevented from eating any 'ordinary' dairy products. The parents of each child would need to give permission and be actively involved, but could not be permitted to know whether their beautiful and initially healthy baby was getting the A1 or A2 formula. This is called a 'blind trial' and it is a very important element of experimental design. Indeed to have a high level of scientific validity the trial should be 'double blind', where none of the scientists dealing with the babies, nor their parents, nor the investigators doing the blood analyses, would know which baby was receiving which treatment. Someone totally separate would hold the codes. (These, and other principles of scientific investigation, are discussed in more detail in Appendix 1.)

It is therefore not surprising that scientists often seek out easier methods of getting answers than by working directly with human patients. One such approach is epidemiology: looking at what happens to populations of people over time in regard to disease incidence, or alternatively looking at different populations at a point in time. (In medical terminology, 'incidence' measures the number of new cases per year; 'prevalence' measures the total number of cases, both new and old, in a population.) Another approach is to use animals as surrogates for people, in the hope that animals will react in the same way as humans.

Bob Elliott decided to look at the problem both ways. The epidemiological approach was to compare the incidence of disease against the intake of A1 and A2 milk for each country. For the animal work he decided to use mice that had been specially bred for susceptibility to diabetes. One of his co-workers in both projects was Dr Jeremy Hill.

The initial results with the mice were exciting. Elliott found that there was indeed a difference in the diabetes incidence between those fed the A1 beta-casein and those fed A2 beta-casein. In fact none of the mice fed A2 beta-casein got diabetes, whereas 47% of those fed A1 beta-casein were diabetic after 250 days. He also found that feeding naloxone with the A1 beta-casein nullified the effect. Naloxone is an opioid antagonist. In other words, it blocks the narcotic effects of opioids. Elliott would have known that if there were a difference between the digested A1 and A2 beta-caseins, it would almost certainly be related to the release of BCM7. He would also have known that BCM7 was a powerful opioid, as this had been published back in 1985.[3] These results therefore suggested very strongly that the effects of the A1 beta-casein were indeed linked to the opioid characteristics of BCM7, although the mechanism by which this might be occurring was not apparent.

Some people might argue that this initial work is best considered as preliminary, in that it was not a 'blind' experiment. In other words, the investigators who did the analyses knew which group of mice was getting which feed. Also, it was not published in the normal scientific literature, but instead as a paper in a special 1997 publication of the International Dairy Federation called *Milk Protein Polymorphism*.[4] Within the scientific community such publications are considered less weighty than international journals. But it did get things started. It provided an empirical (data-based) underpinning of the hypothesis. And it certainly made some people in the dairy industry sit up and take notice.

The other thread of Bob Elliott's work was epidemiology. It was initially thwarted by difficulties in getting data on the A1 and A2 milk composition in different countries. But good fortune intervened at this stage through the chance involvement of Dr Corran McLachlan. Dr McLachlan had been working on processes to manufacture low-cholesterol and cholesterol-free foodstuffs, and was asked by the New Zealand Child Health Research Foundation to review Elliott's 1994 work programme. The Child Health Research Foundation was a Rotary charity set up to fund child-health research. McLachlan was startled when looking at the incidence of Type 1 diabetes to see that the incidence correlated very strongly with data on heart disease with which he was already very familiar (Figure 1).

In a letter to the *New Zealand Medical Journal* in March 2003, in which this graph was published, Corran McLachlan wrote,[5] 'Considering IDDM [Type 1 diabetes] is thought to be a disease of immune stimulation and IHD [ischaemic heart disease] is a disease associated with immune compromisation, the parallels are remarkable. This similarity raises questions with respect to commonality of the source of damage, as well as the time of primary damage.'

In referring to 'the time of primary damage', McLachlan was suggesting that the causal agents of heart disease might be doing their damage early in life, a point which I will come back to in Chapter 3. But the really

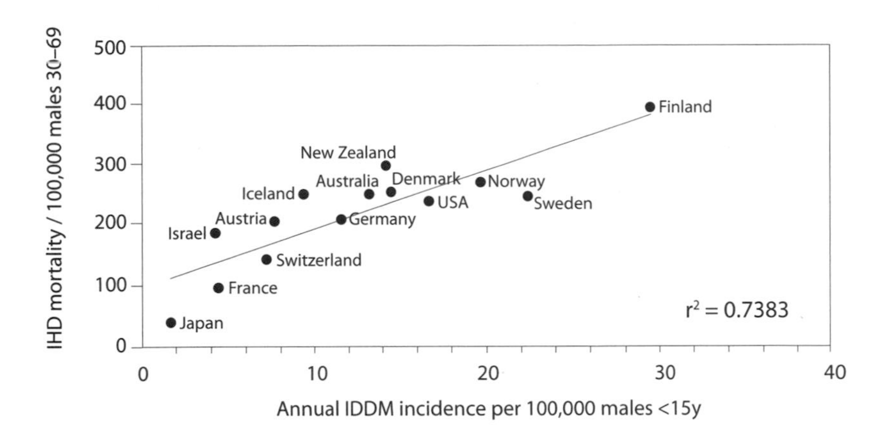

Fig. 1. IHD death rate 1985 for males aged 30–69 vs IDDM incidence for males aged <15. (Reproduced with permission from the *New Zealand Medical Journal* 116 (1170).)

important message was the strong implication that there was a common factor causing both heart disease and Type 1 diabetes. Populations that had high levels of heart disease (mainly among their old people) were the same populations that had high levels of Type 1 diabetes (mainly developing in young people). Statistical theory (which I will turn to in more detail later) tells us that it is highly unlikely that a correlation as strong as this would be simply due to chance. In other words, there is a very high probability of one or more common causal factors.

Determining that countries with high Type 1 diabetes also had high rates of heart disease was a defining moment in the life of Corran McLachlan. It caused him to redirect his own research work. From 1994 until his tragic death from melanoma in August 2003 he was driven by the belief that A1 beta-casein, and the BCM7 fragment that derives from it, were a huge public health issue affecting both heart disease and Type 1 diabetes. It became the focus of both his professional and personal life.

Among the key figures in the story of A2 milk, Corran McLachlan and Bob Elliott stand pre-eminent. So who was Corran McLachlan? The following description is taken from an obituary that was for several years on the A2 Corporation website.

> Corrie McLachlan was born in 1944 to an old established New Zealand family and raised on the family farm in Masterton with his two

brothers and his sister. His country upbringing engendered a love of natural history that remained with him throughout his life.

He was educated at Wairarapa College where he developed his interest in physics and chemistry and also became the head boy and senior athletics champion. In 1962 he went on to Canterbury University where he gained a first class honours degree in Chemical Engineering. This was followed by a move to Cambridge University in England, where he completed a PhD thesis on the Reactions of CO_2 in Alkaline Solutions under Professor de Danckwerts in 1969.

During this time, he met and married his wife, Ulrike, who was working in Cambridge as an au pair. He also began to collect rare books on natural history, later specializing in the natural history of New Zealand.

Dr McLachlan returned to New Zealand in 1970 to take up a position in the Chemistry Division of the DSIR, doing biotechnology research on polymers, agricultural processes, and the dairy industry. He was the recipient of the first United Development Corporation Inventor's Prize in 1974.

After two years as a Visiting Research Fellow at the Engler-Bunte Institute, University of Karlsruhe between 1975–77, Dr McLachlan returned to the DSIR in 1978 as Group Leader of the Industrial Research Division, investigating biotechnology, food processing, industrial chemistry, and chemical engineering.

In 1981 he joined the Energy Section of the NZ Treasury, where he conducted appraisals of the Electricity Division, NZ Power Planning, and NZ Steel.

Dr McLachlan then joined Kupe Group in 1985 as the General Manager, New Investments; and also became an Executive Director of Duncan & Davies Nurseries Ltd, responsible for Operations and Management in New Zealand, as well as Chairman of their UK subsidiary.

Three years later, he set up a venture research company with the Morrinsville-Thames Valley Dairy Co-operative to manufacture a cholesterol-free butter and low-fat meat products through the use of novel extraction technology. He remained as the Managing Director of Tenon Developments Ltd until his death.

Dr McLachlan was made an honorary Senior Research Fellow of the School of Biological Sciences, Auckland University, in 1995. He authored 29 scientific papers and confidential reports and holds 11 patents.

He is survived by his wife, Ulrike, and their three children, Julia, Michael, and Kate.

Clearly, Corran McLachlan was a remarkable man. He was one of those few people who could cross disciplines and make the great leaps needed to advance our understanding about the world we live in. He was also a man of great passion. But he was also a person who could work away painstakingly, putting together the detailed analyses on which the great leaps in knowledge are built. Scientific knowledge seldom advances in a linear fashion. Rather, a range of experiments provide new pieces for the jigsaw puzzle. Inevitably some trials head up blind alleys, and other trials give only partial answers. To get the right answers you have to ask the right questions, but often the right questions are less than obvious at the start.

However, by the start of 2000 the work of McLachlan, combined with the work of Elliott and his team, plus other scientific groups working internationally, was coming together into a big picture. By that time it was evident that the countries with high levels of Type 1 diabetes and heart disease were indeed also the countries that had a high intake of A1 beta-casein. It was also evident that digestion of A1 beta-casein could lead to the release of BCM7, whereas BCM7 was apparently not formed from A2 milk. It was also undeniable that BCM7 was a powerful opioid (narcotic). So the epidemiology, biochemistry and pharmacology were all coming together to tell a powerful story. But the mechanism or mechanisms by which this nasty narcotic might be causing heart disease and Type 1 diabetes, and whether or not it was a common mechanism or separate mechanisms for the two diseases, remained a mystery.

By early 2000 two important patent applications had been filed. The first of these was held jointly by the Child Health Research Foundation (which had supported Bob Elliott's work) and the NZ Dairy Board (the employer of Jeremy Hill, through the NZ Dairy Research Institute, which it fully owned). This patent related to a method of testing milk for A1 beta-casein, which the patent application said was implicated in Type 1 diabetes. The second patent application was by Corran McLachlan and related to the genetic testing of cows for the A1 allele, i.e. testing whether they would produce A1 beta-casein. The patent application claimed that the A1 beta-casein was associated with heart disease.

The next big step in the A1 and A2 milk story began to unfold in February 2000, when McLachlan joined with entrepreneur Howard

Paterson to form the A2 Corporation. Paterson was a larger-than-life figure who was widely considered to be the wealthiest man in the South Island of New Zealand. McLachlan had been searching for months to find a commercial partner. His own funds were running short and he had sold off a precious Goldie painting and a significant proportion of his valuable book collection to keep the work going. He was beginning to despair until introduced to Paterson, who had become New Zealand's biggest agricultural venture capitalist.

Paterson's wealth was largely self-made. He seemed to have a marvellous ability to recognise business opportunities, and always to get his timing right. His early investments were in student flats in the city of Dunedin during the 1970s. At the time he was studying the philosophy and phenomenology of religion for his Bachelor of Arts. In the mid-1980s he left New Zealand for Hawai'i and took his money with him, only to return a few years later when the New Zealand dollar was in the doldrums and New Zealand investments were very cheap.

By 2000 Howard Paterson was New Zealand's and probably the world's biggest dairy farmer. He was certainly the world's biggest deer farmer and New Zealand's biggest egg-producer. He also had diverse investments in property, tourism and wine. He was starting to venture into biotechnology and was in the process of bringing several biotech companies to market. In fact he seemed to have an involvement in just about everything in the South Island of New Zealand that was linked to land. His reputation meant that wherever he went, others followed. As a result, he had got to the stage of being able to stitch together deals whereby he could make a project come together without necessarily investing huge sums himself.

A2 Corporation was just one of four biotech companies that Howard Paterson set up around this time. According to Fiona Rotherham, writing in the magazine *Unlimited* in March 2002:

> Paterson himself paid nothing or virtually nothing for any of his shares in the companies. It is what right-hand man [David] Parker[6] calls 'carried interest' – an American venture-capital term. Paterson's stakes range from 21.5% in Botry Zen to around 15% in Blis and Pharma Zen and 13% in A2 Corporation. He gets the shares dirt cheap in return for bringing in other habitual and retail investors and for his nous in commercialising the products.

In its first year A2 Corporation raised NZ$12.8 million in capital. Initially there was NZ$800,000 from Paterson and his business associates, giving them 65% of the company, with McLachlan owning 35% in return for his intellectual property. Then, towards the end of the year NZ$12 million was raised from institutional and retail investors in return for about 22% of the company. The initial shareholdings of Paterson and his associates dropped to about 48% and McLachlan's shareholding dropped to a little over 30%. With hindsight, those who got in early with Paterson got the best deal. The four directors were Corran McLachlan (who was also Chief Executive Officer, based in Auckland), Howard Paterson (based in Dunedin), Wayne Burtt (a venture capitalist based in Monaco and long-time associate of Paterson's) and Jim Guthrie, a well-known Dunedin lawyer, as Chair. Jim Guthrie had previously worked with Paterson as an adviser on many projects. He was also well known as a former Chair of the Health Research Council of New Zealand, and former Chair of the New Zealand Conservation Authority.

At the end of the March 2001 financial year the company had book assets of about NZ$4 million in cash and another NZ$8.6 million of intangible assets. These intangible assets were mainly the book value (purchase costs) of a 50% share of the diabetes patent that A2 Corporation bought from the Child Health Research Foundation. The McLachlan patent, although now owned by A2 Corporation, did not show up in the books as an asset at this stage. But the market value of the company, as indicated by its share price on the so-called 'Unlisted Exchange', was about NZ$65 million. They were heady days!

In those early days the objectives of A2 Corporation were threefold. First, it had to ensure protection of its intellectual property through patents and trade marks. This intellectual property underpinned the ability to earn royalties from the genetic testing of cows and the sale of A2 milk. Second, it needed to undertake or fund further research that would clarify the role of A1 beta-casein and BCM7 in relation to a number of diseases. And third, it needed to commercialise the marketing of A2 milk through franchise or similar agreements with milk processors and marketers.

Working out how to commercialise A2 milk became a game of intrigue. At that time all of New Zealand's dairy exports were marketed by the NZ Dairy Board. The Dairy Board was a statutory authority owned by the various dairy co-operatives in New Zealand, but also had government representatives on it. Subsequently, the Dairy Board and the two dominant dairy co-operatives were to come together as Fonterra, which now markets more than 95% of New Zealand's milk and about 45% of the world's internationally-traded dairy products. Fonterra also markets a large share of Australia's dairy production through its ownership of Bonlac, Peters and Browne, and major brands such as Mainland cheese, Perfect Italiano, and Cadbury's ice cream. But that was still some time away from happening. So Howard Paterson started talking to Warren Larsen, Chief Executive Officer of the Dairy Board.

Paterson and Larsen were interviewed about their discussions for a March 2003 Four Corners television programme called 'White Mischief'. Four Corners is a long-standing investigative journalism programme screened throughout Australia on publicly-owned ABC television (Channel 2). I have relied extensively on the Four Corners transcript in the following paragraphs.[7]

Howard Paterson's early proposal was that A2 Corporation and the Dairy Board should set up a 50/50 joint-venture company to market A2 milk worldwide. But the talks did not get very far. In fact, Warren Larsen thought that Paterson's proposal was an 'inspirational, novel concept [but] I was certainly not going there'. Paterson's interpretation was that Larsen found his proposal 'outrageous'.

Then in October 2000 Howard Paterson arranged a breakfast meeting with Warren Larsen at the Parkroyal Hotel in Wellington. Paterson gave Larsen a letter suggesting that if the Dairy Board were to ignore the evidence then there was the prospect of a class action by milk consumers at some time in the future. By this, Paterson meant that milk consumers might group together to take court action against Fonterra for supposedly acting irresponsibly. Given Fonterra's international presence, this might take place in a number of countries and according to the specific laws of those countries. Paterson claimed that Larsen's response was to say, 'You can't send this letter to the Board ... I think we need a, um, a collaboration on information.'

Warren Larsen also had a document for Howard Paterson. This document had been written at Larsen's request by Jeremy Hill from the NZDRI. Hill has already featured in this book as Bob Elliott's early collaborator and co-author. At that time the NZDRI was part of the Dairy Board (it later became the Fonterra Research Centre, and more recently part of Fonterra Innovation) so Larsen was Hill's boss. Hill had clearly intended this document to be confidential.

Paterson stated on Four Corners, in relation to Larsen and this document, 'I don't know if he'd read it. I think if he had read it he certainly would not have given it to me. I mean, it's an extremely damaging document to Fonterra.' Larsen's response was: 'I had certainly read it. In fact I am a little bit insulted to think that he would expect me to go to a meeting like that and not have read it.'

Hill's document has subsequently come into the public arena, having been released by A2 Corporation when relationships between A2 Corporation and Fonterra broke down completely. It is long, so here I quote only some key sections. However, the complete document is hugely important and provides further insights into beliefs and attitudes within what was then the NZ Dairy Board, so it is printed in full in Appendix 2.

The overall concern within the document was evident in some early paragraphs:

> If the media (or A2 Corporation) were ever able to assemble the information shown in this paper they could put an alarmist spin on the whole area of milk consumption or alternatively leap to conclusions about A1 vs A2 effects before a case is proven either way.
>
> Taken in totality the contents of this briefing paper could form the basis of an argument for the production of A2 milks and milk products for at risk individuals. However, who may be at risk is still unclear and a diagnostic or diagnostics is a priority. The presence of beta-casomorphin-7 in urine holds some hope in this respect.

Jeremy Hill explained his early involvement:

> The background to this whole area originates from a phone conversation between Bob Elliott and myself in 1993. Bob had phoned the NZDRI and asked to speak with someone who knew something about cows. Bob told me that he thought that casein might be triggering diabetes and asked me if all cows were the same. Upon finding that diabetes was an auto-immune disease and knowing that beta-casein in milk released an immune reactive peptide and that there was a difference in the sequence of this peptide in beta-casein A1 and A2, I suggested to Bob that there might be a difference in the effect of these types of casein on the development of diabetes, although at the time I thought this to be an extremely long shot.

> Under an NZDB funded project NZDRI supplied A1 and A2 caseins for Elliott to feed to diabetes-prone mice.
>
> Only those mice fed A1 developed diabetes.

In relation to heart disease, Hill stated, 'The scientific validity of A2 Corporation's claims that A1 milk is strongly correlated with heart disease is weak.' The justification for those claims will be explored in detail in Chapter 3.

In relation to autism and schizophrenia he said, 'There is growing evidence, but yet unproven that peptides released from milk may be related to occurrence of some mental disorders.'

He further reported that:

> ... work by a German group showed that the bioactive peptide beta-casomorphin-7 (BCM-7) could only be released from A1 type variants (A1, B and C etc) and not A2 type variants (A2 and A3 etc).
>
> This makes perfect mechanistic sense given the differences between A1 and A2 as the proline at position 67 in the A2 variant makes this bond resistant to hydrolysis by digestive enzymes unlike the histidine at this position in the A1 variant.

So here we have an acknowledgement that the empirical facts are consistent with biochemical theory.

Hill also reported on follow-up work on Type 1 diabetes:

> To further investigate if Bob Elliott's feeding trial results could be duplicated a large NZDB funded multi-laboratory multi-national trial was performed – the Food and Diabetes (FAD) Trial. In this trial coded diets supplied from the NZDRI were fed to diabetes-prone rats and mice in Auckland (Elliott), Canada and the UK. Groups in Italy, Germany, and the US also collaborated in the trial.
>
> The effects observed by Elliott were not consistently repeated in the FAD Trial and in fact were shown in only one case, in rats in the Canadian laboratory.

There were multiple misfortunes that befell these trials that might explain this result, including all of the Auckland rodents either dying or having to be destroyed because of bacterial infection. But the really important information lay in some comments that followed about a Mead Johnson product, the hypoallergenic infant formula Pregestimil.

> Another important result from the trial was that [Pregestimil] also produced high levels of diabetes. NZDRI has since shown that Pregestimil contains a high amount of BCM-7. This result is not known outside the NZ dairy industry and forms the basis of a confidential NZDRI Report.

Why were these comments so important? The answer lies in the fact that Pregestimil had been added to half of both the A1 and A2 diets. The presence of BCM7 in the Pregestimil meant that these treatments had been confounded. In other words, here was a trial based on the hypothesis that if there were a difference between the A1 and A2 diets then it would be because of BCM7 released from A1 beta-casein. But *both* diets contained BCM7. What a shambles!

Although Hill acknowledged the Pregestimil issue, he did not make explicit in this memo that it was present in the A2 diets. And in the subsequently published paper, where the presence of Pregestimil was acknowledged, there was no mention that this resulted in BCM7 contamination.

I believe this is a huge issue which strikes at the core of scientific integrity. The trial has repeatedly been used as evidence against the A2 hypothesis by some of the scientists who were involved, without disclosure of the confounding. I discuss this issue in detail, including the steps I have taken to bring it into the open, in Chapter 6.

Hill had more to say about autism and schizophrenia:

> NZDRI has shown that there is a relationship between the consumption of A1 and deaths due to mental disorders. This is only based on epidemiology, but might be possible if BCM-7 affects brain function as suggested by the US work with rats....
>
> There has been circumstantial evidence that the removal of milk and gluten-containing cereals from the diet can reduce or alleviate the symptoms of autism in some children.
>
> A recent patent by a US company has shown that in two thirds of autistic children examined, BCM7 and the equivalent peptides from gluten could be found in their urine but not in the urine from normal individuals.

Hill was also very confident that the NZ Dairy Board's own patents were the key ones, and would crowd out any A2 Corporation patents:

> The claim that A2 Corporation can get around the NZDB patent position is very doubtful.
>
> A2 Corp. claim that the NZDB patent position does not cover the genotyping of animals or the selection of animals for segregation.
>
> The NZDB patent specifically covers genotyping (typing from DNA) and phenotyping (typing from milk).
>
> The NZDB patent is also very comprehensive with respect to the selection of animals and we have discussed this many times with Doug Calhoun from A J Park to make sure that we have not left any loopholes. There are no loopholes and we are sure that the patent could be defended in court.

Fonterra (as subsequent holder of the NZ Dairy Board patents) did indeed oppose A2 Corporation's patent applications, and Jeremy Hill was a key witness. Fonterra's arguments included not only that the science was unsound but also that Corran McLachlan was not the original inventor. On 4 July 2005 the Intellectual Property Office of New Zealand ruled comprehensively against Fonterra and in favour of A2 Corporation on all matters in dispute. Quite simply, Hill's statement that 'there are no loopholes and we are sure that the patent could be defended in court' was proven to be wrong.

From October 2000 onwards the relationship between A2 Corporation and what was to become Fonterra, unraveled rapidly. There was a lot of polarisation. It seemed as if Fonterra staff started taking any opportunity to denigrate the A2 hypothesis. Also, Corran McLachlan in particular started to ruffle plenty of feathers within Fonterra.

One question that people often ask me is why should Fonterra oppose A2 milk? The reasons are complex but they are encapsulated in a quote from Warren Larsen on the Four Corners programme:

> There's one thing in marketing you always need to understand. You never do anything that destroys the category. Nothing. And in this case, that's precisely what the A2 Corporation, in my view, has done.

Stripping aside the marketing jargon, what Larsen meant was that promoting A2 milk would have to be done in a way that did not destroy the overall market for milk. A2 milk would therefore need to be marketed in a way that did not cast doubts on A1 milk! Clearly that would be a challenge!

The reason Warren Larsen argued this way is that although it is not particularly difficult for farmers to change their herds over to being A2 milk producers, it does take time. In fact it takes about two cow generations of breeding, and this means about 10 years. (I will talk more about the breeding strategies in Chapter 10.) The important point here in relation to 'destroying the category' is that while such a change in the herds is occurring, dairy companies such as Fonterra still have to sell a huge amount of A1 milk. So from a dairy company's perspective it would be much easier if A1 milk were a non-issue. And once A2 Corporation started arguing that A1 milk was a health issue, rather than just saying that A2 milk had special positive attributes, then the knives were out on both sides.

But things were to take an interesting turn when, in September 2001, Fonterra applied for another patent, this time claiming that A1 beta-casein was associated with deaths from mental illnesses in general, and in particular was strongly associated with autism. The title of their patent application was 'Milk containing beta-casein with proline at position 67 does not aggravate neurological disorders.'[8] In lay language that means that A2 milk does not make mental disorders worse.

The Abstract for the application then says:

> The invention is based on the discovery that consumption of milk which contains a β-casein variant which has histidine or any other amino acid not proline at position 67, may on digestion cause the release of an opioid which may induce or aggravate a neurological/mental disorder such as autism or Asperger's syndrome. The invention is supplying milk or milk products that contain β-casein with proline at position 67 to susceptible individuals.

In lay language this says that milk containing A1 beta-casein induces or aggravates the symptoms of mental disorders such as autism, whereas A2 milk does not. The patent application then goes on to provide the evidence for these statements. One component is epidemiology from 10 countries showing that intake of A1 milk correlates very closely with World Health Organisation (WHO) data on the level of deaths from mental disorders in those countries. A second component is data confirming that BCM7 is released by digestion of only A1 milk, and not A2 milk. The third is trial data showing that a proportion of autistic children fed A1 milk excreted high levels of BCM7 in their urine whereas ordinary children did not. In contrast, neither autistic nor ordinary children excreted BCM7 in their urine when fed A2 milk.

None of this NZDRI evidence has ever been published in the scientific literature, and subsequently the NZDRI abandoned this patent application, saying that it was unable to replicate the results. Why did this happen? How could this happen? I will have much more to say in Chapter 8 about both this patent application and the subsequent trials, including some enlightening discussions that I have held with one of the researchers.

Meanwhile, a flow of information was starting to appear in the scientific journals. First there was an extremely important paper by Corran McLachlan, published in 2001 in the journal *Medical Hypotheses*. Some Fonterra scientists have tried to denigrate this paper by saying that papers in this journal are not peer reviewed, but this is incorrect. However, one thing that is unusual about *Medical Hypotheses* is that the review process is not anonymous, and it is led by the journal editor who selects apparently worthy papers. Authors know who has made judgements on their papers, and this can have an important influence on the power relationships between author and reviewer. Given that reviewers are often the people with established reputations in a field, they can hold powerful positions that prevent new and competing ideas seeing the light of day. Indeed, many scientists find that they have considerable difficulty getting work published that questions established thinking. In contrast, *Medical Hypotheses* encourages new ideas. And it encourages openness. I have been advised that McLachlan's paper was reviewed by a Nobel Prize winner.

The paper presented statistical data showing a very strong relationship across countries between the level of A1 beta-casein consumption and heart disease, whereas there was no such relationship between A2 beta-casein and heart disease. It also presented data showing a similarly strong link with Type 1 diabetes. McLachlan also pointed out that people such as the Masai and Samburu people of Kenya are 'essentially free' of heart disease despite having very high milk consumption. In both cases the milk they drink is 100% A2. The highest level of heart disease at the time of this analysis was in Finland, where there is a very high intake of A1 beta-casein. France, with mainly A2 cows, has a low level of heart disease. But McLachlan's argument was not based just on words. He presented statistical data showing that the correlations were so high that they were extremely unlikely to be due to chance. He also presented arguments and data suggesting that the method of pasteurisation might be important. And he observed that the long-held medical view that patients with stomach ulcers should be treated with a high-milk diet (the Sippy and similar diets) had been eventually rejected based on overwhelming evidence that it caused heart disease. Were the stomach ulcers allowing the BCM7 easy passage into the bloodstream?

The next important paper was written jointly by Dr Murray Laugesen and Professor Bob Elliott, and was published in the *New Zealand Medical Journal* in early 2003. They presented results of epidemiological investigations looking not only at the relationship between milk and heart disease, and milk and diabetes, but also at all sorts of other dietary factors such as alcohol, fish, meat and vegetables. They showed that there was no other obvious dietary factor that could provide anywhere near the level of association that existed for A1 beta-casein.

The third pivotal paper was one published in September 2003 in the journal *Atherosclerosis* and authored by a team led by Professor Julie Campbell from the University of Queensland in Australia.[9] This paper reported trial work where rabbits were fed a diet containing high amounts of either A1 or A2 milk, and concluded that 'Beta-casein A1 is atherogenic compared with Beta-casein A2.' In lay terms, 'atherogenic' means that it causes heart disease.

All three of these papers will be discussed in more detail in Chapters 3, 4 and 5.

The fourth pivotal paper – or more correctly a stream of papers – came from the work of Professor Robert Cade and his team at University of Florida. Cade's team had been publishing a number of papers showing a link between BCM7 and the symptoms of autism. They knew that the BCM7 came from milk, but not being protein biochemists, they had not known that BCM7 came only from A1 milk and its close variants, and not from A2 milk. It was a classic case of scientists working in different but related fields and not knowing anything about each other's work. But it was not only Cade's team who had evidence that the symptoms of autism were linked to BCM7 from milk. Paul Shattock from Sunderland University in the UK and Professor Kalle Reichelt from Norway had also been working in this field for many years. And of course it all tied in with the Fonterra patent about autism.

So now a much bigger picture was starting to emerge, with BCM7 associated with a whole range of diseases. But there was even more to come. Searching the literature reveals that BCM7 has been identified as a possible factor in sudden infant death syndrome ('cot death'). Also, milk and A1 beta-casein seem to be intertwined with symptoms of Crohn's and similar diseases in some sufferers. Furthermore, milk has been identified as a possible factor in multiple sclerosis, with BCM7 once again standing out as a possible villain.

The one feature that nearly all of these diseases have in common is that they are complex conditions related to the auto-immune system. Another common thread is what is known by the remarkably apt but easily misunderstood name of 'leaky gut'. This does not refer to an unfortunate case of diarrhoea, but a permeable intestine that lets partly digested proteins, called peptides, pass into the bloodstream. No-one is claiming that milk and BCM7 are the simple or sole causes of these diseases. But it does look as if the BCM7 devil could be part of the story.

From 2002 onwards the relationship between Fonterra and A2 Corporation got really nasty. Fonterra scientists presented a paper at the New Zealand Animal Production Society Conference arguing that the work of McLachlan was flawed.[10] Then there was a whole series of papers at the 2003 International Dairy Federation Conference with the common theme of disputing evidence for the A2 hypothesis. But the nastiness was also spilling over into legal action. A2 Corporation took Fonterra to court, arguing that it should be required to put a health warning on all milk containing A1 beta-casein. And Fonterra took A2 Corporation to court, arguing that the recently introduced A2 milk called 'Just A2' involved false advertising because the product supposedly had a level of A1 contamination.

And then things really fell apart for A2 Corporation with the sudden death of Howard Paterson on 1 July 2003 at the age of 50. Paterson was in Fiji for a business meeting but failed to turn up. When his hotel room was checked he was found dead. The autopsy showed that he had choked on some chips. People who knew Howard Paterson tell me it was typical of him to wolf down his meal while concentrating on something else. Somehow a chip lodged in his windpipe and he became unconscious. Death would have quickly followed. Conspiracy theorists have had a range of bizarre explanations as to his death, and who might benefit from it, but the reality is much simpler. He did indeed choke on a chip.

But that wasn't the end of the disaster. By now Corran McLachlan was fighting a losing battle with cancer. He had developed a melanoma ten years or so earlier and it had suddenly returned as secondary tumours in his back. He died in early August 2003, but had effectively been off the scene for quite a few weeks before that.

Ticky Fullerton from the Four Corners programme posted an obituary on the ABC website for these two men, both of whom were larger-than-life figures. About Corran McLachlan she wrote:

> In the short time my producer Quentin McDermott and I spent with Corrie, we were struck by the relentless energy he had to achieve his goal. It was a huge goal: convincing the world, from the housewife to powerful internationals, that a type of milk was the key to better health and that a radical change should be made to dairy herds worldwide.
>
> Corrie McLachlan had a focus that would be hard to match. He used it to great effect in marshalling research to further the A2 cause and battling with the big end of town to get the voice of A2 Corporation heard. Corrie also had a certain eccentricity, which goes with genius, at times awesome, at times hard to keep up with! We remember well how absorbed he became as he shared with us some of his most precious books, stuffed with beautiful watercolours of birds in Auckland ... It is very sad both for Corrie and his family that he will not be around see to how the research on A2 develops and how the story spreads both nationally and internationally.

And about Howard Paterson she wrote:

> Corrie's great supporter, Howard Paterson, lived up to all that we had heard about him: retiring, quixotic, generous and passionate about the many causes behind which he had put his considerable personal and financial support, from farming to education. He was a character ... It was with great pride that Howard showed us over his dairy empire and then with equal fascination and urgency, walked me through the marvelous new university library in Dunedin ... From time to time on a Four Corners shoot, there is the opportunity to spend just enough time with people that they leave a lasting impression. In the case of Corrie McLachlan and Howard Paterson, it was a very good impression. Both Corrie and Howard will be missed greatly in many places.

The deaths of these men could have been the end of A2 Corporation, and they almost were. The company was involved in expensive litigation and running short of cash. As long as Howard Paterson was around, there were further funding options available. But without him the Paterson empire was a different creature. And without the intellectual and emotional commitment of Corran McLachlan there was another huge gap to fill. In fact the company did restructure and live to fight another day under new leadership. But that part of the story can wait. First we need to look in more detail at the arguments for and against BCM7 and some of its truncated forms.

On the surface it might seem that this next part of the story is going to be about science, medicine and statistics. Well, it is. But much of it is also about the people and the games of intrigue that they play.

NOTES

1 Readers familiar with the principles of Linnaean nomenclature will note that the binomial nomenclature used here would seem to denote different species rather than different subspecies. Originally it was Linnaeus himself who used this particular nomenclature and described them as separate species. Although it is now generally accepted that they are best considered as subspecies the binomial (rather than a trinomial) terminology has been retained in general usage.

2 See Cattle Genetics section of Bibliography, in particular Ng-Kwai-Hang and Grosclaude (2002). Although the timing of the mutation is unclear, there is no dispute over chronological ordering of the various mutations, nor that the A2 variant was the original form of beta-casein.

3 See Koch *et al* (1985) in Milk and Casomorphins section of Bibliography.

4 See Elliott *et al* (1997) in Diabetes section of Bibliography.

5 McLachlan CNS.2003.Setting the record straight; A1 beta-casein, heart disease and diabetes. *New Zealand Medical Journal* 116(1170).

6 This is the same David Parker who in 2002 entered the New Zealand Parliament, and then in 2005 became a Cabinet Minister in the New Zealand Government.

7 Australian Broadcasting Corporation. 2003. *White Mischief.* Available at www.abc.net.au/4corners/content/2003/transcripts/s820943.htm

8 See patent application by New Zealand Dairy Research Institute (2001) in Autism and Schizophrenia section of Bibliography.

9 See paper by Tailford *et al* (2003) in Heart Disease section of Bibliography.

10 See paper by Hill *et al* (2002) in Heart Disease section of Bibliography.

CHAPTER TWO

MILK AND CASOMORPHINS

Most readers of this book will not be scientists. And for those who have studied science, it was probably at high school and long-since forgotten. However, in many spheres of life some knowledge of science is very helpful. If nothing else, it helps stop con-artists and rip-off merchants from pulling the wool over our eyes. Or to use another agricultural term, it is helpful in sorting the wheat from the chaff.

In this chapter I want to provide just enough science so that lay people can understand the basic scientific issues that underpin the A2 milk hypothesis. You should not need any existing science knowledge for this chapter to make sense. Indeed it is not necessary to remember all of the facts presented here. But for those with inquisitive minds who want to test the scientific logic of what I say in later chapters, it is in this chapter that the foundations are laid.

Bovine milk (milk from cattle) is about 87% water and 13% 'solids' – fat, protein, lactose (milk sugar) and minerals (Diagram 1). However, there are some differences between individual cows and breeds. For example Holstein/Friesian[1] cows produce milk that is about 12% solids, whereas Jersey milk is about 15% solids.

The protein is of two general types, casein and whey. The casein proteins are the ones that precipitate out in acids, whereas the whey proteins stay in solution. When Little Miss Muffet was eating her curds and whey, the curds contained the casein proteins that had precipitated out as solids. The whey proteins were still in solution as a liquid. So even the term 'solids' is a bit confusing. What we really mean by solids is the non-water part of the milk. If all the water is evaporated off then the solids are what we have left.

The casein proteins can be further divided into three types, these being alpha-, beta- and kappa-casein. In a litre of bovine milk there are

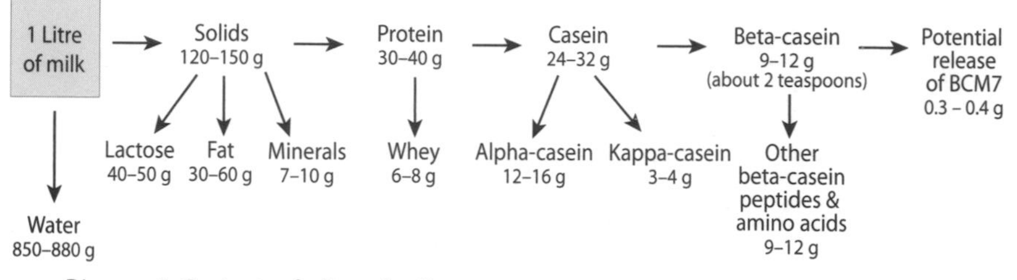

Diagram 1. Contents of a litre of milk.

9–12 grams (about two teaspoons) of beta-casein, again depending on the breed of cow. It is these beta-casein proteins that we are interested in.

All proteins are composed of amino acids. A key characteristic of an amino acid is that it contains at least one atom of nitrogen. Just like fats and carbohydrates (including sugars), amino acids also contain carbon, hydrogen and oxygen. But it is the nitrogen and its binding to hydrogen and carbon atoms that sets amino acids apart. Amino acids are a fundamental building block of life.

According to most textbooks there are 20 amino acids that are found in human tissues. Eight of these are typically classed as essential dietary components, although for infants and possibly old people there can be 10 that need to be ingested. The remainder can be made internally from other amino acids.

When we eat foods containing protein our body breaks down the protein with the help of digestive enzymes produced in our stomach and intestines, first into protein fragments called peptides, and then into individual amino acids. This process is called hydrolysis (*hydro* = water, *lysis* = breaking down), because molecules of water are broken down by reacting with the proteins and peptides. The amino acids that form are then absorbed into the bloodstream. But not all peptides get broken down into amino acids and absorbed. Some are excreted in faeces, and some manage to get through the gut wall into the bloodstream while still in peptide form.

The beta-casein protein that we are interested in here is a folded chain of 209 amino acids. There are at least eight variants of this beta-casein. Initially they were categorised as A, B, C, D, E and F, reflecting the order in which they were identified. Subsequently, the A beta-casein was subdivided into three types, now known as A1, A2 and A3.

In fact it is now known that the most common forms of beta-casein are A1 and A2. The first of these to be identified by scientists was called

A1 beta-casein. A2 beta-casein got that name because it was the second of the A variants to be identified. It was only later that science was able to show that A2 beta-casein was the original one.[2] The only difference between A1 and A2 beta-caseins is the amino acid at position 67 (Diagram 2). In the case of A1 beta-casein the amino acid at position 67 is histidine, whereas with A2 beta-casein it is the amino acid proline.

It may seem surprising, but this tiny difference in the protein structure can have a major effect when the protein is digested. The reason is that

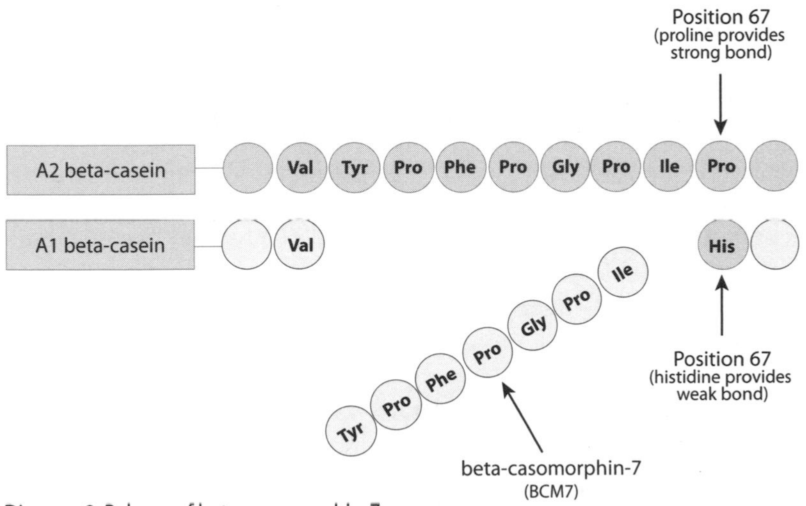

Diagram 2. Release of beta-casomorphin-7.

the proline binds very closely to the amino acid next to it in position 66, which is isoleucine, whereas the histidine linkage with isoleucine is easily broken by digestive enzymes. With A2 beta-casein the proline also binds very tightly with the amino acid in position 68. The outcome of all this is that digestion of A1 beta-casein can produce a peptide of a string of seven amino acids called beta-casomorphin-7 (or BCM7) whereas the evidence is that this does not occur (or at least not to any significant degree) with A2 beta-casein.[3]

The distinguishing characteristics of casomorphins are that they derive from casein and they have opioid (narcotic) properties. Hence the *caso* from casein and the *morphin*, which like 'morphine' derives from Morphus, the Greek god of sleep. The existence of casomorphins and their narcotic properties was first reported in 1979 by German scientists.[4]

The full structure of bovine BCM7 is tyrosine-proline-phenylalanine-proline-glycine-proline-isoleucine. In the shorthand of chemistry this is usually written as Tyr-Pro-Phe-Pro-Gly-Pro-Ile. Fortunately there is no need to remember either the longhand or shorthand version to understand what follows. However, what is important is that the bonds linking the prolines to the other amino acids are particularly strong, and this gives BCM7 great resistance to further breakdown. My biochemist mates tell me that having three proline molecules so close together is very unusual and indeed surprising. But surprising or not, there is no doubt that for cows' milk this is the way it is.

Bovine BCM7 is not the only opioid that can be produced in milk. But it would seem that BCM7, and even more so the BCM5 that can in some situations be formed from it, are by far the strongest.[5] There are also opioid antagonists in milk that can to a large extent negate the effect of the weaker opioids.

In theory it might seem that BCM7 could be formed from A2 milk as well as from A1 milk. After all, there is the same sequence of seven amino acids in both beta-casein variants. It is just the next amino acid along the chain, to which this peptide is bound, that is different (proline instead of histidine). Both Japanese and German scientists have reported in scientific papers that they could not get any release of BCM7 from A2 beta-casein.[6] And, as Jeremy Hill said in the October 2000 document to Warren Larsen that was discussed in Chapter 1, this 'makes perfect mechanistic sense'. This is because the bonds linking this proline to the adjacent amino acids are very strong.

New Zealand Dairy Research Institute scientists (subsequently part of Fonterra Innovation) reported, as part of their 2001 patent application linking A1 milk to autism and related mental diseases, that they too had investigated whether any BCM7 could be released from A2 milk.[7] They reported very small amounts of BCM7 but thought this was likely to be due to some low-level contamination with A1 milk. They concluded that 'if BCM7 was released from the hydrolysis of A2 casein, the rate of reaction was many orders of magnitude less than for A1 casein.'

So it seems that at least on this point there is not much controversy. Scientists essentially agree on where BCM7 does and does not come from, though it would be dangerous to say unequivocally that it is impossible for BCM7 to be released in tiny amounts from A2 milk. This is because digestion is a thermodynamic process and there are random elements to it. But if it does sometimes occur then the amount is very small. In contrast, the amount released from A1 milk can be very large.

So far I have only described the A1 and A2 beta-caseins. But there are also at least six minor variants of beta-casein called A3, B, C, D, E and F. Variants B, C and F all have histidine at position 67 and therefore can be expected to break down just like A1. In contrast, variants A3, D and E all have proline at position 67 and therefore behave the same as A2 in relation to BCM7 release. So when we talk about A1 beta-casein this is really shorthand for the family of variants that act the same as A1. And when we talk of A2 it is shorthand for the family of variants that act like A2.

There are considerable insights to be gained by comparing bovine milk to human milk. As a starting point, it is a fairly safe assumption that if there are problems associated with bovine milk then they will be because of components that are present in bovine milk but absent from human milk, or alternatively because the balance between components is substantially different between the two.

All mammals raise their young on milk but the chemical and physical structure varies greatly between species. To take some obvious differences, whereas bovine milk is only about 13% solids, the milk of polar bears is about 43% solids and grey seal's milk about 68%. Human milk, like bovine milk, is at the watery end of the spectrum: about 13% solids.

Accordingly, the important differences between human and bovine milk relate not to the overall solids content (which is similar for both) but to their constituents. Human milk is higher in lactose, similar in fat, but much lower in protein than bovine milk. It is also considerably lower in minerals such as calcium, sodium and potassium.[8]

I am going to focus here on the protein differences between human and bovine milk. This is not only because the BCM7 story is about proteins (there is absolutely no way that BCM7 could be released from fats, lactose or minerals), but also because most allergies to milk, particularly in children, are associated with its proteins. Many adult humans, particularly those of non-European ancestry, are also intolerant of lactose because they lack the digestive enzyme lactase. But that is another story, albeit a story that may well be relevant to A2 milk, and which I will take up in Chapter 9.

The protein level of human milk is about 1.6% in the first few days following birth and then drops to about 0.9%.[9] In comparison, bovine milk is typically 3–4%, depending on both the breed and individual differences. The specific balance between the proteins is also quite different. In bovine milk about 80% of the proteins are casein proteins whereas in humans the major proteins are whey proteins.[10]

Although beta-casein is the most important of the human casein proteins it is different to the beta-casein produced by cows. The human beta-casein is a shorter protein chain and so the analogous positions in relation to the bovine BCM7 are from 51 to 57 instead of 60 to 66. However, all human beta-casein is of the A2 type rather than the A1 type, in that the adjacent amino acid at the next position (58 in humans and 67 in cows) is proline. This acts as a major barrier to the production of BCM7 in humans.

There is also another extremely important qualification that needs to be made. BCM7 from human milk is not the same as bovine BCM7. In chemical terms it has the structure Tyr-Pro-Phe-Val-Glu-Pro-Ile. In other words, although still meeting the definition of a casomorphin, it has two amino acids that are different from bovine BCM7. A proline and a glycine have been replaced by a valine and a glutamine.

Does this all really matter? Well, yes it does, for two reasons. The first is that the opioid properties of human BCM7 are about ten times weaker than the bovine form. I will return to that later. The second reason is that human milk also releases much less BCM7. Fonterra scientists (led by Jeremy Hill) in association with a Massey University scientist have tested human milk from 15 volunteers to see if they could get a release of BCM7 from it. They stated in a poster paper to the International Dairy Federation Conference in 2003 that on average they got about 2.5 micrograms of BCM7 per millilitre.[11] This is less than 1% of the BCM7 that could be released from the same amount of A1 milk (although they did not make this comparison). So overall, when it comes to the relative opioid effect, human milk has less than one-thousandth the potential potency of A1 cows' milk.

The 'big picture' from this is that human milk is most like A2. It is intriguing that there is this small BCM7 release, and it links with another stream of research that suggests that psychosis in new mothers is linked to their being poisoned either by their own or bovine milk. But that is another story, and beyond the scope of this book.[12]

To get back to the implications for the A2 hypothesis, Jeremy Hill's team have made two claims. The first was that 'these results show that it is likely that some BCM7 is released during the digestion of human milk in the gastrointestinal system.' I have no argument with that, except for the need to make it clear that this is human BCM7 – different to bovine BCM7 – and that it is a very small amount.

The second conclusion was that 'The proposal by McLachlan (2001) that it is the release of BCM7 from beta-casein A1 that makes the consumption of milk containing this variant a risk to human health looks to be unfounded in light of the likelihood that human milks also release an equivalent peptide upon digestion.' I believe this requires a huge leap of logic, given that we have just seen that human milk releases a different casomorphin and in much smaller quantities. Quite simply, Hill's conclusion is totally unsupported by the evidence.

Such a conclusion is highly unlikely to ever be acceptable in a refereed paper, but it is the sort of thing authors can write in a non-refereed poster paper. At this particular conference the attendees were senior staff of dairy companies from all around the world. The vast majority of them would have looked at the conclusions and accepted them at face value. The paper would have reinforced a widespread assumption (which at that stage I myself shared) that the A2 arguments were shonky and misguided. And it would have made the work of A2 Corporation, which was desperately seeking commercial partners from the dairy marketing world, just that little bit harder.

Whether these results will ever appear in the scientific press is unclear. In March 2004 I wrote to the Massey University co-author Dr Alison Darragh (who subsequently became a Fonterra employee) saying that I had seen a comment in an industry magazine, attributed to Jeremy Hill, that the paper was at press. Darragh replied, 'We have published it in abstract form at a conference, and I am currently writing the paper. I will keep your email on file and forward a copy to you when it is published.'

So far I have heard nothing despite a reminder email to Dr Darragh in early 2007, sent to her Fonterra address. I also asked Jeremy Hill himself in March 2007. He said he would follow it up with Alison Darragh as to what had happened, but I have heard nothing. Also, there is no evidence of publication in the international databases, which is a sure sign there is nothing in the peer-reviewed medical literature. But my guess is that if the work does get published (which it should be), the anti-A2 conclusions will be omitted (because the faulty logic would be picked up by the reviewers). However, the damage has already been done. And arguably the industry article saying that the paper was 'at press' (implying that it had been accepted following refereeing by scientific peers) was less than accurate. All that had been written was an abstract.

We can gain some further insights about A1 beta-casein versus A2 beta-casein by looking at the situation with other mammals that are closely related to cattle. What we find is that goats' milk contains A2 beta-casein and no A1 beta-casein. In most, but probably not all sheep, the milk contains only A2 beta-casein.[13] Yaks produce only A2 beta-casein. And so do all *Bos indicus* cattle, which are the native cattle of Asia.

Putting all of this evidence together allows us to say with high confidence that the A2 beta-casein was the original beta-casein, and that in genetic and historical terms the A1 beta-casein is a 'Johny-come-lately'. The most likely time of the mutation of the gene responsible, which is known to be on the sixth chromosome, is between 5000 and 10,000 years ago, at a time when cattle were being taken north into Europe and long before most of the modern European breeds developed.

I am often asked why the A1 variant (or allele) has become so common. Does this mean that the A1 beta-casein has advantages that led to its being selected for, so that it became widely spread throughout European cattle? The answer is probably 'no', since no-one has been able to suggest a likely advantage of A1 beta-casein. The answer is more likely to be found in what animal-breeding scientists call the 'founder effect'.

The founder effect is about the very large impact of the genetic profile of the individual animal from which a breed is founded. For example, a particular bull may have had a superior temperament as a result of a genetic difference that had nothing to do with whether it was A1 or A2. This bull would then have been selected to mate with a range of cows, and the progeny that inherited the same characteristic would then be used to mate with other animals, eventually creating a new breed. If that original bull happened by chance to also be carrying the A1 allele then the animal breeders would unwittingly have been selecting this allele at the same time, so it would become widespread and common throughout the new breed.

The founder effect also answers the other question I am often asked, which is why does the incidence of the A1 allele vary so much between the different modern breeds? Modern breeds have developed within only the last 2000 years, and in many cases over a much shorter period. If, say, the original black-and-white animal happened to have the A1 allele, then the black-and-white breeds would have a high incidence of that allele (and they do). Similarly, if the mutation that led to yellow cattle first occurred in an individual carrying the A2 allele, then it would be expected that the yellow breeds would probably be high carriers of the A2 allele (and they are).

The message from this is that the A1 beta-casein that we find in the milk of so many of our modern cows is essentially an anomaly. The 'original' milk was clearly A2 milk, and the A1 milk that so many of our modern cows produce is probably just an aberration.

But there are other interesting possibilities. For example, we don't know very much about how calves metabolise BCM7. A common effect of opioids is to make animals more placid. Did farmers actively select the more placid calves, and was this placidity caused by drinking opioid-laced milk?

Processed products

So far, when talking about the release of BCM7 from cows' milk, I have been talking about fresh milk. What happens when the milk is processed, producing pasteurised milk, cheese, yoghurt, butter, ice cream and dairy desserts? For some of those products we have some answers, but there remain plenty of unknowns.

First, let's look at pasteurisation – heating milk to kill bacteria. There is a range of pasteurisation methods, ranging from the old Holder method of heating it to about 63°C for about 30 minutes, to the ultra-high-temperature (UHT) method where the milk is heated to 145°C for just a few seconds. There are also intermediate methods such as heating to 90°C for about 15 seconds. In parts of Europe much of the milk is UHT. One of the advantages is that it can be kept unrefrigerated for months as long as it remains sealed. Not everyone likes UHT milk and some people say it tastes different. In the USA, Australia and New Zealand most milk is pasteurised using one of the intermediate methods.

All pasteurisation methods, and indeed any treatment of milk at more than about 48°C, have the potential to break down or denature the protein. Once the key temperature of about 48°C is reached then it is probably the time that it remains heated, rather than further increases in temperature, that becomes critical, although both time and temperature are undoubtedly relevant. As the protein structure breaks down it is unclear which peptides will be released, but in Chapter 3 I will discuss some circumstantial evidence that when milk is pasteurised by the Holder method, more BCM7 may be released upon subsequent digestion than occurs with the intermediate temperature methods.

When making ice cream, milk is commonly heated not just to pasteurise it, but because it becomes much easier to mix with the other ingredients. Hence, according to the textbooks it is common to hold the milk at 70°C for at least 15 minutes. I don't know whether all ice-cream makers do this, but two have confirmed to me that they do. What effect this has on the release of BCM7 is unknown, but there is anecdotal evidence that some people can tolerate ice cream made from A2 milk whereas they get severe diarrhoea with ordinary ice cream. So there is a fair chance that BCM7 may be released from ice cream made from 'ordinary' milk. Whether or not the heat treatment process is important is unclear.

The Fonterra Research Centre (now Fonterra Innovation) has done some interesting work looking at the release of BCM7 in a range of cheeses made from 'ordinary' milk (containing both A1 and A2 beta-casein). Its researchers have shown that the amount released varies greatly, depending on the type of cheese. In mozzarella they found no detectable BCM7; in cheddar they found very small amounts, and in blue vein somewhat more. By my calculations this means that the yield of BCM7 in blue vein was about 1% of the amount that would be formed if all the beta-casein had broken down to release BCM7, whereas in cheddar it was about 0.05%. But this is only the BCM7 released during the cheesemaking process. There is still the question of what additional BCM7 is released during digestion, in the stomach and intestines. The Fonterra data indicate that only 7% of the beta-casein remains intact in blue-vein cheese, so there may not be much more BCM7 that can be released (unless it is in an intermediate form between beta-casein and BCM7). But in contrast, with cheddar 63% of the beta-casein is still intact, and for mozzarella the figure is 69%. What happens when this is digested? Quite simply, we do not know. So how we should interpret all of this information is far from clear.

Anecdotal evidence about intolerance to dairy products suggests that at least some people who cannot tolerate ordinary milk, but can drink A2 milk, can also tolerate moderate amounts of cheese. But the significance of this gets complicated because cheese is also lower in lactose than the milk it is made from. Perhaps more importantly, the epidemiological evidence in Chapters 3 and 5 tends to support the perspective that cheese derived from ordinary milk is not implicated in diabetes and heart disease. In addition, some of my biochemist friends tell me that there are good scientific reasons why the cheesemaking process *might* make the BCM7 inactive. So I'm fairly relaxed about eating cheese made from ordinary milk, but accept that in doing so I am probably still picking up small quantities of BCM7. But I would probably have a different attitude if I thought I was a leaky gut sufferer (which I will soon discuss) and therefore at particular risk of developing one of the auto-immune diseases.

Clearly the issue of BCM7 and cheese is an area where a lot more research needs to be done. So far Fonterra's research in this area has been published only in poster form, first at the 2003 International Dairy Federation Conference, then in the *Australian Journal of Dairy Technology*.[14] Hopefully, at some stage this will be published as a full scientific paper in a peer-reviewed journal. But I am not holding my breath. And is anyone doing some follow-up work? I may be wrong but I think not. No-one has put their hand up to say they are working on it.

What happens to BCM7 in yoghurt is unknown. I cannot find any information in the scientific literature about this. Perhaps it will be a similar story to cheese. But then perhaps not. Without trials all we have is conjecture.

Both sides in the A2 milk controversy seem to agree that BCM7 is not a particular issue in butter. This is because butter is mainly fat rather than protein. Whereas milk contains fat and protein in a ratio of approximately 1:1, in butter the ratio is about 80:1. So unless someone was eating huge amounts of butter, it would not be the source of much BCM7.

Absorption from the Gut

The next important question is what happens to BCM7 when it is released into the gut. Once again there is no simple answer. In healthy adults it should be difficult for BCM7 to get through the gut wall and into the bloodstream, because the molecule is too large. But it appears there are plenty of exceptions. Almost certainly, it depends on the age, health and genetic makeup of the particular person.

Some people suffer from leaky gut syndrome, whereby BCM7 and other peptides pass very easily into the bloodstream. A more formal term is 'intestinal permeability' although it is the former term that seems to be used more widely. And the term 'gut' is arguably more accurate as it encompasses both the stomach and intestines.

In people with a leaky gut it is possible to detect BCM7 in the urine. This condition has been closely associated with the symptoms of autism by Professor Robert Cade and his team from the University of Florida and will be discussed in detail in Chapter 8. There is also very strong circumstantial evidence that people with stomach ulcers or untreated coeliac disease absorb BCM7 through the gut wall. It is also likely that babies can absorb BCM7 the same way; in fact newborn babies need to be able to pass large molecules through the gut wall. Otherwise they would not be able to absorb the colostrum in their mothers' milk. All of this will be discussed in Chapters 8 and 9.

One of Professor Cade's co-workers, Dr Zhongjie Sun, has experimentally injected BCM7 into rats. He and colleagues have published evidence that once in the bloodstream the BCM7 passes very readily across the blood/brain barrier and that it attaches there to opioid receptors.[15] They have also shown that the rats then exhibit behavioural tendencies very similar to those of autism and schizophrenia.[16] They found that the effects could be reversed with administration of naloxone, a well-recognised morphine antagonist. Other scientists have found that BCM7 causes apnoea (breathing dysfunction) in adult rats and newborn rabbits that is analogous to sudden infant death syndrome in humans.[17]

Those of you who sometimes drink the sports drink Gatorade can take some comfort from the thought that you have been a contributor to the work of Professor Cade, Dr Sun and their co-workers. It was Professor Cade who designed the formula for Gatorade, and it is the subsequent royalties (managed by a foundation) that have supported their work into autism and BCM7.

The effects of BCM7 are not restricted to behavioural symptoms. The fact that opioids affect a wide range of immune functions has been known for over a hundred years. This immune effect provides a possible explanation as to why BCM7 appears to be implicated in such a wide range of auto-immune diseases.

However, not all of the effects of BCM7 are necessarily due to its opioid characteristics. The tyrosine molecule on the end of the BCM7, combined with the stability of BCM7, gives the milk devil strong oxidant properties. Indeed BCM7 has been shown *in vitro* (i.e. in a test tube) to be a strong oxidant of low-density lipoprotein (LDL, the 'bad' type of cholesterol).[18] Oxidation of LDL is fundamental to the process whereby fatty plaques are laid down in artery walls, leading in turn to heart disease.[19] So it seems likely that the effect of BCM7 on heart disease may be twofold, with an opioid related mechanism (perhaps linked to immune function) and the oxidant properties working like a double-edged sword.

The BCM7 that is released in the gut can affect the digestive system without necessarily being absorbed into the bloodstream. It is well known that casein is sometimes effective in treating diarrhoea, and indeed can lead to constipation. It is also well known that opioids, including BCM7, can reduce the rate of passage through the gut.[20] For example, a common side-effect of codeine, which is an opioid, is constipation. This may explain why babies fed on milk-formula products rather than human milk are susceptible to constipation and in extreme cases can suffer anal fissures.[21] It is also possible, but at this stage unproven, that the slower passage of A1 milk through the digestive system (due to release of BCM7), increases problems of lactose intolerance. The reasoning here would be that lactose intolerance is due to lactose fermentation caused by the absence of the lactase enzyme, and the slower the passage, the more fermentation will occur.

In summary, it is clear is that there is a lot that we know but also much that we don't know about BCM7. We know that BCM7 is produced from A1 beta-casein but not produced, or produced only in very small amounts, from A2 milk. We also know that BCM7 is a very powerful opioid if it gets into the bloodstream. We know that in some people BCM7 can pass from the gut into the bloodstream, and in animals at least, it then readily passes across the blood/brain barrier. We also have strong evidence that BCM7 can compromise the immune system (I will elaborate on this in later chapters). We also know that *in vitro* BCM7 strongly oxidises low-density lipoprotein, and that *in vivo* (i.e. in the body) oxidation of LDL leads to heart disease.

All this is like a big jigsaw puzzle, where the overall picture is starting to appear, or indeed, arguably, is already clear. But there are still plenty of small pieces to come. This is not surprising, because scientific puzzles rarely come together in a straightforward way. Prior to Bob Elliott's discussions with Jeremy Hill back in 1993 no-one had even thought of A1 beta-casein as being the culprit. So it is a work in progress. Nevertheless, the big picture seems to be clear: BCM7 really is a little devil. Little in the sense of size, but very big in terms of the mischief it can cause.

I will have more to say about BCM7 as this book progresses. But for the meantime enough has been said, and it is time to start looking at some of the diseases linked to the milk devil.

NOTES

1 Holstein and Friesian are both black and white breeds. They are sometimes regarded as the same breed.

2 See Ng-Kwai-Hang and Grosclaude (2002) in Cattle Genetics section of Bibliography.

3 See Hartwig *et al* (1997) and Jinsmaa and Yoshikawa (1999) in Milk and Casomorphins section of Bibliography.

4 See Henschen *et al* (1979) and Brantl and Teschemacher (1979) in Milk and Casomorphins section of Bibliography.

5 There is a range of milk peptides that have these opioid characteristics. These casomorphins always have a tyrosine molecule as the amino acid at one end, and a particular type of amino acid known as an aromatic amino acid, such as phenylalanine or another tyrosine, in either the third or fourth position on the chain. The presence of proline in position two is crucial for the biological activity of the casomorphin, as it maintains the proper orientation of the tyrosine and phenylalanine side chains. How many other amino acids are hanging on the chain will also have some modifying influence on the bio-active properties of the particular casomorphin.

6 See Hartwig *et al* (1997) and Jinsmaa and Yoshikawa (1999) in Milk and Casomorphins section of Bibliography.

7 See New Zealand Dairy Research Institute (2001) in Autism and Schizophrenia section of Bibliography.

8 It is inevitable, given that human milk is high in lactose, that it is also low in minerals. This is the only way that the milk, while in the mammary glands, can be iso-osmotic with blood.

9 These figures come from the Australian National Health and Medical Research Council's 2003 publication *Dietary Guidelines for Children and Adolescents in Australia*. Other references commonly list the protein level as about 1.1%. However, there are considerable inconsistencies in the published literature on human milk, and it is impossible to rationalise some of the stated figures for total protein, casein percentage, and beta-casein.

10 Most of the proteins in human milk are whey proteins but in general these are not the same whey proteins as in cows' milk. Human milk has no beta-lactoglobulin, which is the major whey protein in bovine milk, and bovine milk has only very small amounts of lactoferrin, a major whey protein in humans. This lactoferrin is believed to be important in human milk as a protective factor because of its anti-bacterial properties.

11 See Norris, Darragh *et al* (2003) in the Milk and Casomorphins section of the Bibliography

12 See Lindstrom *et al* (1990) in the Milk and Casomorphins section of the Bibliography.

13 The NZDRI reported in its subsequently abandoned 2001 patent application relating to autism and schizophrenia that the SWISSPROT database recorded some sheep as having an alanine at position 67. This alanine could be expected to act in the same way as a histidine and hence these sheep could be expected to produce BCM7.

14 See Norris, Coker *et al* (2003) in Milk and Casomorphins section of Bibliography.

15 See Sun, Cade, Fregly and Privette (1999) in Autism and Schizophrenia section of Bibliography.

16 See Sun and Cade (1999) in Autism and Schizophrenia section of Bibliography.

17 See Hedner and Hedner (1987) in Milk and Casomorphins section of Bibliography.

18 See papers by Steinerova *et al* in Heart Disease section of Bibliography. Also the paper by Torreilles and Guerin (1995) – but beware, this is in French.

19 The modern view of heart disease is that inflammation of the arteries and the heart muscle is also a key factor. It is this inflammation, which is itself an immune response, that allows the deposition of fatty plaque to occur. This is because the surface of an inflamed artery is rough and sticky rather than smooth. For a detailed but eminently readable review see the article by Peter Libby in *Scientific American*, May 2002, pp. 47–55.

20 See Becker *et al* (1990) and Defilippi *et al* (1995) in Milk and Casomorphin section of the Bibliography.

21 See Andiran *et al* (2003) in Milk and Casomorphins section of Bibliography.

CHAPTER THREE

POPULATION STUDIES OF HEART DISEASE

There are three parts to the evidence that A1 beta-casein is linked to heart disease. The first is evidence that countries where people have high intakes of A1 beta-casein, also have a high incidence of heart disease. This is called epidemiological evidence. The second part is trials involving animals and humans, in particular a trial in which rabbits fed A1 beta-casein developed arterial plaque, whereas rabbits fed A2 beta-casein did not. The third part is pharmacological evidence showing how the BCM7 that derives from A1 beta-casein is linked to oxidation of low-density lipoprotein (LDL), which in turn causes arterial plaque. I will look at these in turn. In this, the first of two chapters on heart disease, the focus is on the epidemiology.

There is more than one type of heart disease and the United Nations World Health Organisation (WHO) has a considerable number of subcategories. Most of the analyses reported here are for ischaemic (or coronary) heart disease, which is by far the most common form of heart disease. It is caused by build-up of fat deposits on the artery walls, leading eventually to a blockage. Often this occurs when a piece of plaque breaks loose from elsewhere and blocks the coronary artery that supplies blood to the heart muscle itself. The blockage cuts off the supply of blood, damaging the muscle and causing what we call a heart attack. Throughout this chapter, when I use the term 'heart disease' I am referring specifically to death from this type of heart disease. On other occasions I use slightly broader terms, such as cardiovascular deaths, where the authors I am quoting have used those terms.

The first indication that A1 beta-casein was related to heart disease came about quite by chance. In 1994 Dr Corran McLachlan was asked by the New Zealand Child Health Research Foundation to review Professor Bob Elliott's work programme. The Child Health Foundation is an independent charity set up and supported by Rotary, and to which scientists can apply for support. Bob Elliott was reporting initial work and seeking further research funds to investigate the link between A1 beta-casein and Type 1 diabetes. The normal procedure is that such applications and reports are forwarded to one or more independent scientists to assess their merit. This process is known as 'peer review'.

When Corran McLachlan looked at Bob Elliott's data showing how the incidence of Type 1 diabetes varied between countries, he was struck by the amazing correlation between the incidence of Type 1 diabetes in various countries and the incidence of heart disease in these same countries. At this time Elliott knew there were enormous differences in the incidence of diabetes between different countries (up to 300-fold) and McLachlan knew that there were very large differences in the incidence of heart disease between different countries (about fourfold). But scientists tend to work in isolation from other scientists working in different fields. There is so much to read and to do, that diabetes researchers don't normally read the work of heart-disease researchers, and vice versa. So it came as a great shock to McLachlan to see that there was this remarkable relationship.

The graph that McLachlan obtained when he plotted out the data linking diabetes and heart disease has already been shown in Chapter 1 (Figure 1, p. 19). In statistical terminology, McLachlan obtained an r^2 value of 0.74, meaning that 74% of the variation in the incidence of one disease could be explained by the variation in the incidence of the other disease. If there had been no relationship between the two disease levels then the r^2 value would have been 0. If there had been perfect correlation such that the points for the different countries lay exactly on a straight line then the r^2 value would have been 1. Anyone who knows anything about biology and statistics will immediately recognise that for cross-sectional data an r^2 value of 0.74 is remarkably high and indicates a very strong correlation. But scientists and statisticians are also very cautious about how such relationships should be interpreted.

One of the first lessons about correlation is that it doesn't necessarily mean that there is a causal link. It could be that the relationship is just by chance, or it could be that both variables (diabetes and heart disease) are influenced by a third variable that the scientists have not identified. For example, there is an extremely strong relationship between breast cancer and the wearing of dresses. But that does not mean that wearing dresses causes breast cancer. Similarly, people who get prostate cancer tend to be people who wear trousers. In both cases there is a third factor, that of gender, which is the causative factor.

People who study statistical relationships are called statisticians. Statisticians who specialise in biological data are often called biometricians. And biometricians who specialise in disease incidence (either human or animal) are called epidemiologists.

One of the first tests a statistician does with data such as these is to investigate whether or not the relationship is 'significant'. In using the term 'significant' statisticians are not asking 'Is it important?' Rather, what they are asking is whether or not it is likely to have been caused by chance. In other words, is it a random or fluke result, or is it something we can rely on? Surprisingly, McLachlan never presented the results of this statistical test. But it is an easy test for a high-school or undergraduate student with access to the appropriate statistical tables to do, and shows that the chance of getting this result purely by chance, or through a fluke of the data, is less than one in a thousand. (For those who understand the language of statistics, the correlation, which has 15 degrees of freedom, is significant at $p < 0.001$.) This is a mind-blowing result. We can therefore be very confident that it is not just due to chance.

So what does it mean? That one disease is causing the other? No: heart disease is mainly a disease of adults, whereas Type 1 diabetes usually shows up in childhood. Therefore heart disease can't be causing the diabetes. Further, many more people get heart disease than Type 1 diabetes. Therefore it seems very unlikely that the Type 1 diabetes could be the major cause of heart disease.

What this correlation is telling us very clearly is that there is a hidden factor, or several factors acting together, that cause *both* heart disease and Type 1 diabetes. These factors must clearly include a factor or factors that are environmental rather than genetic, because all ethnic groups have higher incidences in high-risk countries than in the low risk countries. So it must be something in the physical environment, or else it must be something in what people eat and drink.

By this stage Bob Elliott already had some evidence to suggest that A1 beta-casein was indeed a key factor in Type 1 diabetes. He had some early results of trials with mice, and he also had some early indications that there were strong correlations between countries with a high incidence of Type 1 diabetes and countries with high A1 beta-casein intake. But this epidemiology data also had limitations owing to uncertainty at this early stage about the true levels of A1 beta-casein intake in various countries.

Until this time there had been only minor interest in the different types of protein in cows' milk. Dairy scientists had shown some interest but it had not attracted any attention from health scientists. Those dairy scientists who had recognised that different breeds of cows had different levels of the various proteins, including differences in the incidence of A1 and A2 beta-caseins, had seen no need to put all the data together in terms of national and regional differences.

At this time Corran McLachlan was running a company researching the production of cholesterol-free dairy and meat products. Indeed he already had a patent on the production of cholesterol-free butter, but he was less than convinced that it was the answer to reducing heart disease, and he was searching for other answers. As part of this work he had put together a research file on foods associated with coronary heart disease. One of these files covered milk proteins and pasteurisation. McLachlan was sufficiently impressed by what he was seeing that he devoted the next five years of his life to documenting the intake of A1 and A2 beta-caseins in different countries.

Aspects of McLachlan's research were first brought into the public arena with his 1996 patent application for genetic selection of cows to eliminate A1 beta-casein in milk, and thereby reduce the incidence of heart disease. But hardly anyone reads patent applications except patent lawyers. Patent applications are made as early as possible, as it is critically important to be the first to make a particular claim. There is a fine line to getting in early enough to gain precedence while also being convincing in the claims being made. Some of the crossing of the scientific t's and dotting of scientific i's comes later. So the key paper is McLachlan's 2001 publication in the international journal *Medical Hypotheses* by which time most of the wrinkles in the argument against A1 milk had been ironed out (Figure 4).

The data on heart-disease levels that McLachlan used came from the WHO studies of age-standardised data for a range of countries. Two data sets were available, one for 1985 and the other for 1990. Both were for death rates from coronary heart disease in males and females (considered separately) aged 35–69 years. The data on total milk consumption came from the United Nations Food and Agriculture Organisation (FAO). The data on A1 beta-casein and A2 beta-casein for each country came from a range of published sources. For each country, a two-stage process was used. First, information was sought on the prevalence of the A1 beta-casein allele in the various breeds of dairy cattle in each country, and then this prevalence was weighted by the importance of each breed in the national herd. McLachlan was able to find data for 17 developed countries, including 12 European countries plus Canada, the USA, Australia, New Zealand and Israel.

The results he obtained were remarkable. He found that the correlation between total dairy protein consumption and the incidence of male deaths from cardiovascular disease was quite weak, with an r^2 of 0.26. When he looked at the relationship between the deaths and A2 beta-casein consumption it was even weaker, with an r^2 of 0.16. However, the correlation between coronary heart disease and A1 beta-casein consumption was exceptionally high, at 0.71. When McLachlan excluded the A1 beta-casein from cheese consumption, the r^2 value increased even further to 0.86 for male death rates in 1985 and 0.84 for the death rates in 1990. The justification for excluding cheese consumption from the analysis was based on theoretical (but not proven) evidence that the release of BCM7 is much lower from cheese than fresh milk. (Aspects of this were discussed in Chapter 2.) Female death rates followed a similar pattern, though with slightly lower r^2 values.

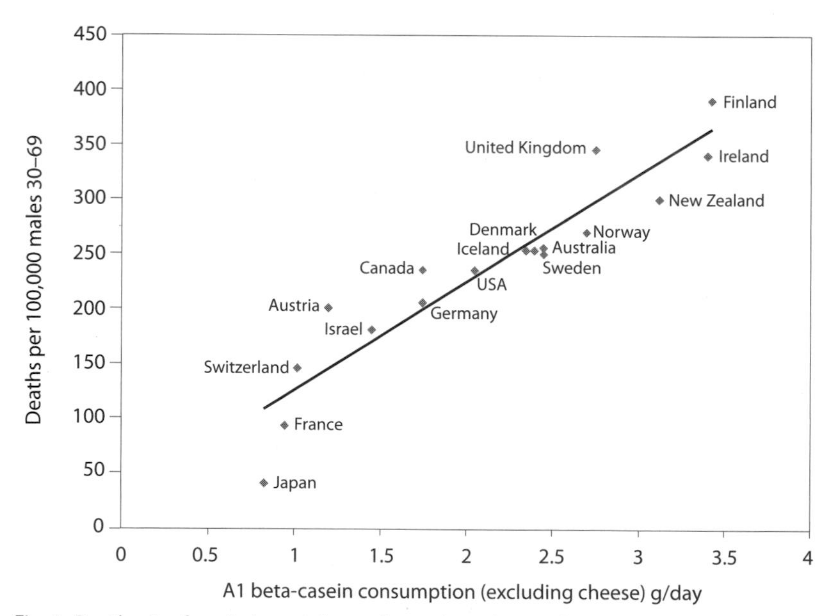

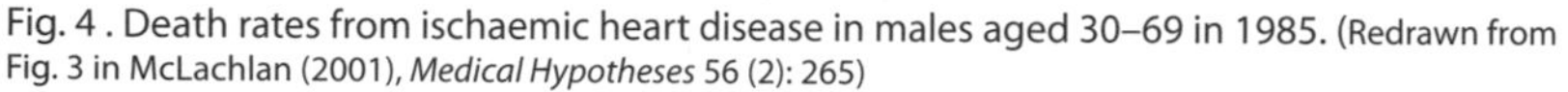
Fig. 4 . Death rates from ischaemic heart disease in males aged 30–69 in 1985. (Redrawn from Fig. 3 in McLachlan (2001), *Medical Hypotheses* 56 (2): 265)

The statistical tests show that the probability of getting chance or fluke results such as this, whereby the incidence of cardiovascular deaths can be explained to this extent by intake of A1 beta-casein, is less than one in a thousand for both males and females. Effectively, we can cast aside the possibility of this result occurring by chance. That leaves three alternatives. The first is that the data have been 'cooked', either accidentally or purposefully, to give either an erroneous and perhaps even fraudulent result. I will put aside that possibility in the meantime, but will return to it shortly. The second possibility is that A1 beta-casein is indeed a major risk factor leading to heart disease. The third possibility is that there is some other factor yet to be identified that is correlated to A1 beta-casein that is causing the problem. In other words, that people who live in countries where a lot of A1 beta-casein is consumed are also subjected to some other factor that not only causes heart disease but also in some way affects intake of A1 beta-casein, whereas people in countries consuming low amounts of A1 beta-casein are not exposed to that other factor, whatever it might be.

The best way to explore each of these possibilities is to look at another paper, this time by Dr Murray Laugesen and Bob Elliott, that was published in the *New Zealand Medical Journal* in January 2003.[1] Whereas Corran McLachlan's paper is painted on a broad canvas and is breathtaking in terms of its picture, the Laugesen and Elliott paper makes much heavier reading. It is carefully structured and contains more detail as to exactly how the data were obtained, and these data are presented in a form that enables others like me to do our own calculations to test what Laugesen and Elliott have done. As a consequence it is not light reading, but as I have read it again and again I have come to appreciate that it is an extremely professional and objective piece of research.

Murray Laugesen is a researcher with Health New Zealand. According to the Health New Zealand website (www.healthnz.co.nz):

> Dr Murray Laugesen founded Health New Zealand as his consultancy company in 1995, after 18 years in the Department, then Ministry of Health, and Public Health Commission. Since 1995, Dr Laugesen has shifted focus gradually from tobacco policy work to tobacco control research, but with the same aims – to reduce cancer, heart disease and smoking; and create a smokefree New Zealand.

Murray Laugesen holds many awards, including a WHO medal 'for achievements deemed worthy of international recognition in promoting the concept of tobacco-free societies', and a Queen's Service Order for public services. Laugesen has particular strengths in public health and epidemiology. In conversations with other medical researchers who know him, I have received the consistent message that he is very methodical and fastidious. He is much more likely to get things right than wrong, and it is not often that his work is criticised by other scientists.

The first criterion Laugesen and Elliott used when selecting countries was whether or not published data on A1 beta-casein levels were available. This criterion was met by 23 countries. The next criterion was whether annual expenditure on health care was at least US$1000 per person based on purchasing-power parities. This criterion was important to prevent introducing bias between poor and wealthy countries. Hungary and Venezuela were excluded on these grounds. In addition, the Netherlands was excluded because of simultaneous high imports and exports of dairy products and the consequent inability to determine the origin of milk consumed. This selection process meant that the sample comprised 20 of the world's 22 'health affluent' countries.

As well as investigating the relationship between coronary heart disease and A1 beta-casein, Laugesen and Elliott also used FAO food-supply tables to investigate the intakes of 77 other food types, and 110 other measures of nutritional intakes. The purpose of these analyses was to search for any other factors that could be affecting disease incidence.

The correlation coefficients that Laugesen and Elliott measured, based on A1 beta-casein intake and heart disease mortalities in 1980, 1985, 1990 and 1995, were all extremely high and all were significant at the level of $p < 0.001$. This means that the probability of getting results like this by chance is in each case less than one chance in one thousand. Laugesen and Elliott also found evidence that the intakes of wine, vegetables and polyunsaturated fats from plants are each associated with lower levels of heart disease, but the relationships were considerably weaker than for A1 beta-casein. There was no consistent relationship between heart disease and the amount of tobacco products smoked. (This is an interesting side-issue that I take up later in this chapter.) And the relationship between A1 beta-casein and heart disease was much stronger than the relationship between heart disease and estimated average serum cholesterol levels for inhabitants of these countries, as measured by what is called the Hegsted score.

Taken in totality, the Laugesen and Elliott evidence seems very clear.

There is an incredibly strong relationship between the amount of A1 beta-casein consumed and the level of heart disease. There is also evidence that other factors like wine drinking and intake of polyunsaturated fats from vegetables may be important. But there is no other factor out there that gives anywhere near the explanation that A1 beta-casein does. So if the differences in disease levels really are due to some factor other than A1 beta-casein, then it remains a total mystery as to what that could be. We can say with a high degree of confidence that it is not a factor such as wine drinking or intake of polyunsaturated fats. The reality is that the culprit would seem to be staring us in the face: it's A1 beta-casein.

What we find is that the McLachlan paper and the Laugesen and Elliott paper are singing the same tune. They have used somewhat different data sets, and relate to somewhat different time periods, but the overall message is the same. It doesn't matter whether the analyses relate to 1980, 1985, 1990 or 1995. Nor does it matter whether the assumed lag between dietary intake and effect on heart disease is five years or ten. Laugesen and Elliott looked at all these possibilities. Nor does it matter whether the analysis is carried out using data just for males (who have a higher incidence of heart disease than females) or for both sexes combined, or even just females. Nor does it matter whether the analyses are for people aged less than 65 or more than 65. Every time the same result comes up: that there is a remarkably strong relationship between intake of A1 beta-casein and coronary heart disease, and we can be very confident that this has not come about by chance.

Despite the common tune of the message coming from both papers, the authors were not exactly mates at this time. Corran McLachlan had been working totally independently of the others. In fact Bob Elliott was somewhat aggrieved that McLachlan had latched onto some of his intellectual property without sufficient acknowledgement. In particular, Elliott believed that the claims McLachlan had made in his initial patent application overlapped with an earlier patent based on his own work. The testiness between them even spilled over into the news media. This would seem to refute any suggestion that the data was in any way 'cooked' or manipulated. Two totally independent studies have come up with the same answers.

Returning to Corran McLachlan's paper again, there is a lot of additional supporting circumstantial evidence for the role of A1 beta-casein that comes from other observations and analyses, but which was not included in the statistical analyses that I have reported so far. For example, McLachlan noted that the Masai and Samburu communities in Kenya drink large amounts of bovine milk but have little or no heart disease; similarly for rural Gambians. In all of these cases the milk they drink comes from non-European cattle and contains little or no A1 beta-casein. Essentially, all of the beta-casein is A2. The story is the same for Tibetan highlanders who drink yak milk, which is also A2.

McLachlan also compared the incidence of heart disease in the various states of West Germany. He found that 66% of the variation in deaths from heart disease could be explained by differences in the level of A1 beta-casein intake, based on the different breeds of cattle found in each state. Because there are only eight states, the correlation required for statistical significance was higher than for the other analyses. However, these results are significant at the 2% level ($p< 0.02$). This means that the likelihood of getting such a result by chance is less than one in fifty.

McLachlan also discussed the results of a study comparing the incidence of deaths from heart disease in Belfast and Toulouse. This work was undertaken by the Northern Ireland and French centres involved with the MONICA study, a major survey undertaken by the World Health Authority on cardiovascular death rates and the associated risk factors. The death rates from heart disease in Belfast were three to four times those in Toulouse, despite all the classical risk factors being, to use McLachlan's words, 'virtually identical'. About the only difference of note is that the citizens of Toulouse tend to drink more wine than the citizens of Belfast, who imbibe similar amounts of alcohol, but in drinks other than wine. McLachlan presented data showing that the intake of A1 beta-casein was 2.49 times higher in Belfast than in Toulouse, and observed that in the light of all the other evidence, this is highly suggestive as to what the true factor is.

The possibility that red wine in moderation is good for heart health has gained a lot of credence from studies reporting that the rate of heart disease is considerably lower in Mediterranean countries such as France and Italy than in northern Europe. Almost everyone seems to have heard that a diet containing olive oil and red wine is great for heart health. There is a fair chance that this proposition is correct, and I am more than happy to go along with it as I enjoy my glass of red wine each night with my evening meal. But I am also very aware that the statistical evidence is less than compelling and it may well be a chance relationship. Indeed the statistical evidence associating wine with low heart disease is very much weaker than the evidence associating A1 beta-casein with high heart disease. And it just so happens that these heart-healthy Mediterranean countries also have comparatively low intakes of A1 beta-casein. In part this low intake is because they tend to consume less milk, but also the breeds of cows in these countries have a low prevalence of the allele that causes them to produce A1 beta-casein. And even if we were to accept that red wine and olive oil are reasons for low levels of heart disease in these Mediterranean countries, this does absolutely nothing to explain why the Masai, the Samburu, the Tibetan yak herders and the Japanese all have low incidence of heart disease.

Iceland and Finland provide some more interesting evidence. Ethnically, these Scandinavian peoples are very similar and they have similar diets. However, Finland has one of the highest levels of heart disease in the world, whereas in Iceland the incidence is only about 60% that of Finland. Is it coincidence that the intake of A1 beta-casein in Iceland is also only 60% that of Finland? (This difference in A1 beta-casein intake is because the Norske cows in Iceland have a higher level of A2 beta-casein and a lower level of A1 beta-casein in their milk than the Finnish cows.)

The situation in the Channel Islands south of England is even more interesting. On the island of Guernsey, where the milk comes from the Guernsey breed of cows which produces milk with very low levels of A1 beta-casein, the level of deaths from coronary heart disease is about a third that of the rest of the UK. And in Jersey, the cows are predominantly the Jersey breed which produces milk with some A1 beta-casein, but considerably less than the predominant black and white breeds on the mainland, and the heart disease level is only about half that on the mainland.

One of the fascinating things about heart disease is that the incidence has varied greatly over the last hundred years. Before the 20th century heart disease was only a very minor cause of death, partly because people died of other diseases before getting heart disease. But the story is far from that simple. Age-adjusted data (i.e. that allows for the fact that an increasing proportion of people now live to an age where heart attacks become more likely) show that heart disease increased greatly during the first half of the 20th century. Why was that? Perhaps it was due to lifestyle changes, with many people doing less physical work and starting to lead sedentary lifestyles. But perhaps that is only part of the story.

Equally fascinating is that after reaching a peak in the 1960s, heart disease incidence has been progressively declining. It has not declined to anywhere near the level of the 19th century, and in most developed countries it is still the most important cause of death, but it has gone down markedly. Why this decline should be occurring is also a considerable mystery.

Both the McLachlan and the Laugesen and Elliott papers have pointed out that this decrease cannot be explained by the so-called 'classic' risk factors such as raised serum cholesterol and blood pressure. However, Laugesen and Elliott do make the observation that between 1985 and 1995 heart disease rates declined by 37%, and this was accompanied by a 13% decline in A1 beta-casein consumption.

The counter-attack

A feature of the evidence I have reported so far is that it all points in the same direction. The next question, therefore, is whether or not I have reported all of the evidence. Is there something else out there to take the gloss off the arguments I have presented?

Yes, the epidemiological evidence has been criticised. These criticisms fall into two categories. The first category is that the methods of analysis are basically unsound. The second category is not with the methods or the results themselves, but with how much weight we should give to these results.

Criticisms of the first type appear to have come almost exclusively from within Fonterra, New Zealand's largest dairy co-operative. Fonterra is a major force within the dairy world. It markets over 95% of New Zealand's dairy production, about 40% of Australia's dairy exports, and is also an increasingly important player in the Australian domestic industry. In total, about 45% of the world's internationally traded dairy products come from Fonterra, including in 2006 some 76% of US exports. It exports dairy products to about 150 countries. The size and scope of Fonterra means that it has a considerable scientific research capacity. It also has a very professional public-relations machine.

Fonterra scientists have publicly argued against the A1 epidemiological data in at least three scientific fora. The first was a paper presented at the 2002 annual conference of the New Zealand Society of Animal Production (NZSAP) and subsequently published in the proceedings of that conference.[2] The second was a letter in the *New Zealand Medical Journal* in early 2003.[3] The third was a poster paper at the International Dairy Federation Conference in 2003, subsequently published in the

Australian Journal of Dairy Technology.[4] During 2002 and 2003 Fonterra scientists also took these arguments into the news media.

Papers published in *Proceedings of the New Zealand Society of Animal Production* are only lightly refereed. I know something about this as I have myself been a referee for this publication. Scientists present their research in written form several months before the conference, and unless the written version is incoherent or obviously flawed, it tends to get published. There are tight publication deadlines to ensure that the proceedings are available at the time of the conference. As a result, fellow scientists do not generally regard these as 'full' scientific papers, though they are a very good way of getting a short sharp message across to a professional audience. In the allotted time and space there is no opportunity to present all the details that would be necessary for comprehensive peer review.

The *Australian Journal of Dairy Technology* could at best be described as an obscure journal; in fact the Lincoln University librarians tell me that the only library in New Zealand that seems to subscribe to it is the Fonterra Research Centre. Given its obscurity, it might seem remarkable that some of the arguments presented there get exposed to such a wide audience. But then perhaps it is not so remarkable after all. With a good public-relations system it is not too difficult to get the media to pick up press releases along the lines of 'a recently published scientific paper has found that ...' The news releases do not need to emphasise that it was Fonterra's own scientists who did the research and that there was no or very limited peer review.

The NZSAP paper was published in 2002, after the McLachlan paper but before the Laugesen and Elliott paper. It was authored by three Fonterra research scientists: Jeremy Hill, Robert Crawford and Michael Boland. This is the same Jeremy Hill who collaborated with Bob Elliott in the 1990s on the early work suggesting A1 beta-casein was implicated in diabetes, and in patent applications he was associated with arguments against A1 milk and for A2 milk up until 2001. His name keeps cropping up throughout this book.

The claims that the Fonterra team make in this paper include that

> Epidemiological evidence for a relationship between the consumption of milk (and of beta-casein A1) with heart disease appears to have been a serendipitous correlation that occurred in the past (perhaps due to a common underlying factor) but now no longer holds. Elimination

of beta-casein A1 from the diet will have no effect on the mortality effect due to heart disease.

Well, that all seems very unequivocal and at least we have no doubt as to where they stand on the matter! But how did they come to that conclusion?

What they did was to conduct a correlation analysis for 40 countries (the specific countries are not identified, which is very unusual in a scientific paper) between deaths from coronary heart disease and consumption of total milk protein. What they found was that up until 1991 there was a statistically significant relationship between intake of milk protein and deaths from heart disease. But thereafter the relationship was non-significant. Remember that 'significant' means unlikely to be caused by chance, and that 'non-significant' means we cannot be confident that it was not caused by chance, or what can be described as 'random noise' in the data.

There are three major problems with the Fonterra analysis. Each of the first two problems by itself completely destroys the credibility of the researchers' analysis. The third problem is a level of confounding that is also probably fatal.

The first problem is that they worked with *total* milk-protein intake rather than A1 beta-casein intake. Bob Elliott knew back in the early 1990s that it was not simply milk-protein intake that mattered; indeed that was exactly the reason he first telephoned Jeremy Hill. So a poor data fit does not come as any surprise. In fact Corran McLachlan also got a low correlation when using milk-protein intake. Subsequently, in a letter in the *New Zealand Medical Journal*, Jeremy Hill justified the use of total milk protein rather than A1 on the basis that the two were highly correlated.[5] But this doesn't tell the full story. For example, an analysis that I undertook of the Laugesen and Elliott data shows that only a little more than half ($r^2 = 0.57$) of the between-country variation in A1 beta-casein intake can be explained by intake of dairy protein. It would only have taken Hill five minutes with a spreadsheet to find this out, if he had thought to do so. Furthermore, it is surprising that he was not already well aware of this from analyses that he and others presented in the patent application linking A1 beta-casein to autism and mental illnesses (and discussed in detail in Chapter 8). In those analyses they had found a strong relationship between A1 beta-casein and deaths from mental illness, but only a weak relationship between those deaths and total milk protein. The whole basis of the argument is that disease rates vary between countries not only because of the amount of milk consumed, but because of the different breeds of cattle, and hence different levels of A1 beta-casein in that milk. A heart-disease analysis based on total milk protein as a proxy for A1 beta-casein could be described as total nonsense.

The second problem became evident when I referred to the WHO database to check out the data used in the Fonterra analysis. I found that WHO had subsequently withdrawn the database because it had found that there were anomalies in the most recent years. So that seemed to explain very easily why Fonterra could not find any correlations for those particular years. Quite simply, the data that Fonterra had used had too many holes in it, and the provider of the data had temporarily withdrawn it.[6]

The third problem scarcely needs mention, given that each of the two earlier ones has independently destroyed the Fonterra argument, but I will touch on it in passing. It is that the Fonterra scientists were working with raw data from 40 unidentified countries. To get this number of countries they would have had to select countries with greatly different wealth levels and greatly different health systems. Working with such data is always likely to produce the statistical equivalent of a fog. In contrast, McLachlan focused on developed countries and Laugesen and Elliott focused on 'health affluent' countries to filter out these confounding effects.

Actually, there appears to be a fourth problem which initially escaped me. There is no mention that they have used death rates for a particular age category, or what that age category might be. It appears that their data was for all ages. Using such crude data, countries with higher birth rates over the last 20–30 years than other countries will inevitably, other things being equal, have low overall death rates, for no other reason than the lower average age of the population. Such data would, for example, almost certainly show that some Catholic countries, which were slower to introduce birth control than Protestant countries, had a lower death rate in relation to total population for almost any disease one chose to select. But would that prove that Catholics were healthier? Hardly! In the case of heart disease, such data would inevitably produce a fog.

As a final comment on this paper and where it was published, the standard method of searching for existing medical information is to interrogate the PubMed database, an internet service of the US National Library of Medicine. As of 2007 it contains more than 16 million citations – but it does not include the *Proceedings of the New Zealand Society of Animal Production.* This means that this publication is not the place to publish research on health matters if you want to ensure other health scientists will easily be able to locate and read your work. But it does enable you to say in the news media that you have published relevant research on health matters. However, there is also an argument that the information has not been properly 'published' at all – using the meaning that scientists give to the word 'publish'. The paper itself was a review paper (which means it should not introduce new, unpublished data). So what has happened is that the Fonterra scientists have published their conclusions without ever providing the details of their data for others to scrutinise.

The second part of the Fonterra counter-attack was to argue in the *Australian Journal of Dairy Technology* that by excluding cheese from the analyses the work was fundamentally flawed. The Fonterra scientists (this time C.S. Norris, C.J. Coker, M.J. Boland and Jeremy Hill, with Hill as the corresponding author) questioned whether this was valid because they have shown that there is some BCM7 in cheese (presumably derived from the A1 component).[7] However, they have also shown that the amount of BCM7 obtained is only a very small proportion of the potential release. These results with cheese have already been discussed in Chapter 2. The reality is that there is a lot of what statisticians call cross-correlation or co-variance between the intake of cheese and intake of milk. In other words, countries with high intake of A1 beta-casein from milk also tend to be countries with high intake of A1 beta-casein from cheese. So it is actually quite hard from the epidemiological analyses to say whether cheese intake does or does not relate to heart disease. But the indication from the somewhat higher correlations obtained when cheese is excluded from the analyses is that A1 beta-casein from cheese may not be a major cause of heart disease. The Fonterra research showing that the release of BCM7 from cheese is quite small is consistent with this position. In addition, the fact that the release of BCM7 varies between cheese types suggests that it would require a very sophisticated statistical model to capture the relationship. So although the Fonterra scientists argued to the contrary, the results they obtained from cheese tended to support the work not only of McLachlan, but also of Laugesen and Elliott.

As soon as the Laugesen and Elliott paper was published in the *New Zealand Medical Journal* there was a flurry of letters to the editor. Many journals do not publish letters, but it is not uncommon for medical journals to allow a correspondence to deal with matters of controversy. When this occurs it is a sure sign that the authors of the paper have struck a nerve amongst other researchers. In fact the Laugesen and Elliott paper was sufficiently controversial that an editorial was penned in the same issue, written by Professors Robert Beaglehole from the WHO and Rod Jackson from the University of Auckland. They congratulated Laugesen and Elliott for their work. But they also expressed concern that research into A2 milk should not be at the expense of programmes focusing on known risk factors such as cholesterol, blood pressure and smoking. Communicating this message to the public about these risk factors has been an important focus of their careers.

The Laugesen and Elliott paper also looked at the epidemiology of Type 1 diabetes, and some of the correspondence focused on diabetes. I am leaving that to Chapter 5. However a letter from Jeremy Hill, in his role as General Manager of the Fonterra Research Centre, and published several weeks later in the *New Zealand Medical Journal*, was critical of the whole approach, and needs to be considered in this chapter.[8]

Most of Hill's criticisms can be ignored, in that they were based on conjecture and misunderstanding, and were subsequently demolished when Laugesen and Elliott presented further information in their response.[9] But Hill did make a point in relation to tobacco that is really interesting, even if the correct interpretation of his point is perhaps quite different. He argued that a major criticism of Laugesen and Elliott's work was that they 'could find no relationship between smoking and heart disease, when this is already known to be a significant health factor. The lack of a correlation with tobacco consumption very much highlights the dangers of relying on epidemiological data as evidence of cause and effect.'

Well, the reality is that the evidence linking smoking to heart disease *is* also epidemiological. However, the accepted epidemiology for smoking is based on within-country analyses rather than between-country analyses. According to the website of the American Heart Society (www.americanheart.org), smokers have two to four times the risk of non-smokers of having a heart attack. In contrast, the Laugesen and Elliott analysis, based on between-country comparisons, showed that countries with low smoking rates tended if anything to be the high heart disease countries, and high smoking countries (such as Japan) were often the countries with low rates of heart disease. How could this be?

There are no simple answers to this question, but the Laugesen and Elliott data does show very strongly that smoking is not the reason that heart disease varies so much between countries. Hence the Japanese, who seem to be getting things right in relation to other risk factors (including intake of A1 beta-casein) have remarkably low rates of heart disease despite being heavy smokers. Perhaps they would have even lower heart-disease rates if they smoked less. And maybe many of the people in Japan who do have heart attacks are also smokers. Neither of those possibilities can be denied. But what the Laugesen and Elliott analyses indicate is that although smoking may well be a very important cardiovascular health issue for individuals, at a country level the effects of smoking are being swamped by other factors. *And we need to find those other factors if we want heart disease rates in other countries to decline to rates such as in Japan or even as in France.*

Where Jeremy Hill went astray was to use the apparent lack of association between smoking and heart disease at the country level to discredit the whole approach of between-country epidemiology. I regard this reasoning as fatally flawed. The scientific approach to information such as this should be to reflect and ask: what does this really mean? And what are the insights that flow from this?

The biggest problem with all epidemiology is trying to exclude other factors. For example, smokers tend to exercise less than non-smokers, and arguably are less likely to look after their health in general. If they smoke, then what else do they do that is unhealthy? Sorting out one factor from the others is very difficult, perhaps impossible. Personally I hate smoking and I believe there is no doubt that it is a causative factor in many diseases. But it is indeed fascinating that some countries with a high average level of smoking can also have low rates of heart disease.

Another example that illustrates a similar point about within-country epidemiology is the case of Vitamin E. For a long time it was widely believed that Vitamin E gave very clear health benefits and this was presumed to be because it was acting as an antioxidant. The evidence seemed very clear that people who had been taking Vitamin E supplements had lower incidence of a number of diseases. But then when 'blind' trials were conducted, with some people getting the supplements and others taking a placebo, there was no clear difference in health outcomes. How could this be? Once again there is no definite answer, and there is still debate as to the benefit of Vitamin E. However, the most likely explanation would seem to be that the people who had previously been taking the Vitamin

E were also the sort of people who looked after their health in many other ways related to diet and lifestyle. So benefits attributed initially to Vitamin E were perhaps really due to a multiplicity of factors.

A key point about between-country epidemiology (also called ecological studies) is that, for a factor such as A1 beta-casein, each country is essentially a 'blinded' participant. Neither the countries nor the individuals within those countries made a conscious decision as to whether they would drink milk for which the beta-casein was predominantly A1 or predominantly A2. They weren't offered the choice, or even aware there was a choice: it was a matter of chance, depending on the predominant breeds of cattle in each country. By restricting the analysis to countries that had similar wealth and healthcare systems, it provides a very powerful comparison of like with like.

One point I agree with is that epidemiology by itself can never provide final, absolute proof. But it can provide very strong evidence. And if A1 beta-casein is not the answer then what *are* the causative factors? Laugesen and Elliott have searched methodically but without success for alternative explanations, and so have their detractors. Early in this chapter I used the example of the association between people who wear dresses and people who get breast cancer. It may have seemed a frivolous example, but I actually took it from a newspaper quote attributed to Dr Chris Mallett from Fonterra, who was using it to illustrate the point that an association does not necessarily indicate causation. He then linked that idea to the situation with A1 beta-casein. Fair enough – but why is it that in the case of heart disease and A1 beta-casein no-one can explain what the third factor is? It is simply not good enough to say it is chance, given the nature of the statistical probabilities.

In 2005 a new argument emerged from what might be called 'the Establishment' as to why the A1/A2 epidemiology evidence, as produced by McLachlan, Laugesen and Elliott, was supposedly flawed. The argument was propounded by Professor Stewart Truswell in a paper published in the *European Journal of Clinical Nutrition*,[10] although very similar arguments were being mounted at that time by the Australian dairy-industry group, Dairy Australia. Professor Truswell is a retired professor of human nutrition from Sydney University, who remains professionally active.

Professor Truswell was used by Fonterra as their key external scientific witness in the New Zealand Intellectual Property Office Tribunal hearings in 2004/05 where it was opposing the A2 Corporation genotyping patent. Professor Truswell's task was to rebut the arguments and evidence of A2 Corporation. He was described by Fonterra as 'the senior professor of human nutrition in Australia', and with publications going back to 1957 it is hard to argue against that. However, the Intellectual Property Office did not support Professor Truswell's scientific arguments that included criticisms of the work of McLachlan, Laugesen and Elliott, and dismissed all of Fonterra's claims.

When Truswell's similar arguments were published in the *European Journal of Clinical Nutrition* in May 2005 I responded with a long letter to the editor of that journal. This was published in March 2006. (Everything takes time in the scientific world!) There was also a letter from Dr Andrew Clarke (A2 Corporation's Chief Executive Officer at that time) and Dr Jock Allison (an A2 Corporation director) in the July 2006 issue, together with an author's right of reply from Professor Truswell to both letters. At this point I will focus only on the arguments about epidemiology, although there are other points in Professor Truswell's writings that I will take up in the final chapter.

In essence, Truswell argued that if A1 beta-casein caused heart disease then we should be able to see evidence of this in within-country heart-disease and heart-mortality statistics. People who drank more milk would inevitably have a larger intake of A1 beta-casein, and if A1 beta-casein was harmful they would have more health problems.

There are four problems with this argument. The first problem is to get good data on what people *actually* drink, and to then follow this through for several decades to see what happens to them. The second problem is to isolate all of the associated dietary and lifestyle issues. The third issue is that if damage is being done, we don't actually know when in life it takes place. But in Chapter 4 I will present some evidence that for some people it may be very early in life when the intestines are permeable (or 'leaky') so that large molecules can pass through from the intestine into the bloodstream. I will also present in Chapter 4 some very strong evidence that the damage may take place during any period of life when, for a range of reasons, a person suffers from a leaky gut. Indeed the leaky gut syndrome is a recurring theme throughout this book. The fourth issue is that proponents of the A2 hypothesis are likely to also be very comfortable with the notion that there are good things as well as bad things associated with milk drinking, and that some of these things may be cancelling each other out.

I will illustrate the first two of these problems by referring to a study of what is known as the Caerphilly cohort. The most recent available data are from a paper in the *European Journal of Clinical Nutrition* with Professor Peter Elwood from Cardiff as the senior author.[11] Truswell cites this and similar papers approvingly as part of his argument against the A2 hypothesis.

The Caerphilly study involved approximately 2500 Welsh men born between 1920 and 1935. They entered the study between 1979 and 1983 and have been followed up through to 2003. Their milk intake was based on a questionnaire they filled out at the time of commencing the study, recording 'milk drunk' per day. For a subset of 665 men this was compared to a seven-day record of all milk and milk-product intake (i.e. including milk in all foods consumed as well as actually drunk). The relationship between the data from the seven-day diet records and the data from the questionnaires had an r^2 value of 0.37.[12] In other words, the questionnaire answers captured only 37% of the actual variation in milk intake between people in the study during that seven-day period.

So we have a huge issue to start with in terms of reliability of data! (It was the questionnaire data that was subsequently used for the remainder of the study, although some separate work has been published using the subset data.) And even if the questionnaire had been accurate at the time (which clearly it was not), would it have been accurate for the years that followed? Or for the preceding years, perhaps going right back to early childhood? It is important to recognise that milk intake was not measured again as the study progressed.

The second problem is trying to sort out confounding effects of other lifestyle factors. The men were divided into four milk-drinking categories: non-drinkers, drinking up to half a pint, half to one pint, and more than one pint per day. (A pint equals 0.57 litres). It was found that the non-milk-drinkers also drank more alcohol, were fatter, apparently more sedentary, and had a greater proportion of fat in their diet. They also had higher blood pressure at the outset. So there were huge problems in sorting out what was due to milk (or lack thereof) and what was due to other factors.

Further, although the proportion of men having heart attacks apparently decreased somewhat as milk intake increased (i.e. there was an inverse relationship), these results were not statistically significant. In other words the statistical properties of the data were such that it was impossible to confidently draw any conclusions, even in relation to all of the factors considered together. In simple terms, there was a fog. We cannot say with any confidence that there is either a positive relationship or a negative relationship. And even if there was a positive or negative relationship, we would still have great difficulty deciding which factor or factors were causing it.

And that is the way it is with most of these studies.

The final point in relation to Truswell's argument is that milk may have *both positive and negative* effects. To quote from a presentation Professor Elwood gave in 2005 at a Dairy Australia seminar, 'Drinking milk raises cholesterol levels.'[13] He said that many papers reported this effect – and also that many studies reported a reduction in blood pressure.

We all know that low cholesterol is supposed to be good, and so is low blood pressure. Therefore we seem to have conflicting forces at work here. Also, within the dairy industry there is a huge amount of research underway to identify a range of bio-active components that are beneficial. All that the A2 people are saying is that in among all these good things there also seems to be a little devil.

Pasteurisation

Before leaving the epidemiological evidence it is worth looking briefly at some issues relating to milk pasteurisation.

Corran McLachlan put forward a suggestion in his *Medical Hypotheses* paper that both the historical increase and subsequent decrease in levels of heart disease worldwide might be linked to the method of pasteurisation. He drew together evidence from a range of sources to show that, as pasteurisation of milk was introduced in various countries and regions within countries, within a few years there was a marked increase in the level of heart disease. Prior to 1950 the major method of pasteurisation was the Holder method (the milk was heated to 63°C for about 30 minutes). Subsequently this method fell out of favour, largely because of the distinctive 'cooked' flavour it gave to the milk. In the 1960s there was a move to short-time, high-temperature methods, (about 90°C for 15 seconds) and by 1980 these had become predominant. This change was soon followed by a decline in heart-disease levels that cannot be satisfactorily explained in terms of the classic risk factors for heart disease.

Corran McLachlan was not the first person to put forward the possibility of a link between pasteurisation methods and changing levels of heart disease, but he did take the argument further than previously.

He hypothesised that the heat treatment regime used in the Holder method was leading to protein breakdown and providing an increased level of BCM7 from A1 beta-casein. It's an interesting proposition. The evidence looks quite strong, and it seems to make a lot of sense in terms of what we know about what happens to proteins when they are heated. But more work is required. It would be a marvellous research project for someone so inclined to investigate *in vitro* (i.e. in the test tube) the effect of heating on the subsequent release of BCM7 from A1 beta-casein. And also to test what happens to this milk subsequently when stomach enzymes are added.

So the pasteurisation story is intriguing and may be important. In most countries we no longer use the Holder method of pasteurisation but we still do, for a range of reasons, use heated milk in a number of products. And it is a standard procedure when mixing ice-cream ingredients to heat the milk to a temperature and for a duration that is similar to the Holder method.

Summary

The work of Corran McLachlan, and even more so the work of Laugesen and Elliott, tells us that there are very strong relationships linking intake of A1 beta-casein with heart disease. The relationships are highly significant in a statistical sense and therefore cannot be dismissed as due to chance. Almost certainly the apparent link is a real link. However, we cannot say that these statistical correlations by themselves 'prove' that A1 beta-casein causes heart disease, because no correlation can ever 'prove' causation with *absolute* certainty. But if A1 beta-casein is not causing heart disease, then what is the third factor that causes these extremely strong relationships? No-one has been able to suggest what that might be.

If A1 beta-casein does indeed cause heart disease in humans then it is reasonable to expect that it might also cause heart disease in some animal species. Given that animals are easier to work with in experimental trials, this is an obvious issue to investigate. Also, it would seem reasonable to expect that science might be able to provide at least some pointers as to how the A1 beta-casein and its associated milk devil are doing their damage. It is these issues that will now be explored in Chapter 4.

NOTES

1 See Laugesen and Elliott (2003a) in Heart Disease section of Bibliography.

2 See Hill *et al* (2002) in Heart Disease section of Bibliography.

3 See Hill (2003) in Heart Disease section of Bibliography.

4 See Norris, Coker *et al* (2003) in Milk and Casomorphins section of Bibliography.

5 See Hill (2003) in Heart Disease section of Bibliography.

6 In July 2004 when I was first investigating this issue, the hyperlink that the Fonterra scientists supplied as their data reference led to an explanation of this effect. By March 2005 both the database and the reasons for its withdrawal had disappeared from the WHO website. By early 2006 the database was operative again, presumably with amended data.

7 See Norris, Coker *et al* (2003) in Milk and Casomorphins section of Bibliography.

8 See Hill (2003) in Heart Disease section of Bibliography

9 See Laugesen and Elliott (2003b) in Heart Disease section of Bibliography

10 See Truswell (2005) in Industry, Marketing and Overview section of Bibliography.

11 See Elwood *et al* (2004) in Heart Disease section of the Bibliography.

12 Within the paper itself this was presented as r =.61. For consistency I have converted this to the equivalent r^2 value.

13 Proceedings of the 'Hearty Choice Seminar'. Available at www.dairyaustralia.com.au/content/view/130/188/

CHAPTER FOUR

THE TRIALS AND SCIENCE OF HEART DISEASE

There are three parts to this chapter. First, there are the trials investigating whether animals fed A1 beta-casein are more likely to get heart disease than those fed A2 beta-casein. The second part looks at what we know about the underlying science as to how the milk devil might cause heart disease. The final part looks at the big picture and what the various bits of the jigsaw puzzle seem to be telling us.

The rabbit story: A1 beta-casein is atherogenic

The most important of the animal trials linking A1 beta-casein to heart disease was undertaken at the Centre for Research in Vascular Biology at the School of Biomedical Sciences, University of Queensland. The research was under the direction of Professor Julie Campbell and was published in 2003 in the international journal *Atherosclerosis*. The title of the paper is a very bald statement: 'A casein variant in cow's milk is atherogenic'.

So what do these 'athero' words mean? According to the *Hutchinson Encyclopaedia*, 'atherosclerosis' means 'hardening of the inner lining of the arteries with fatty degeneration'. 'Atherogenic' means 'leading to atheroma'. And 'atheroma' means fatty degeneration of the arteries. *Atherosclerosis* is therefore a journal that publishes research on artery disease. It is published by the leading international scientific publisher Elsevier.

The particular protein variant that this paper refers to is A1 beta-casein. In lay language, the paper is saying that A1 beta-casein causes fatty degeneration of the arteries.

The four authors are listed as Kristy Tailford, Celia Berry, Anita Thomas and Julie Campbell. Professor Campbell is listed as the corresponding author, indicating that the work was directed by her and she is taking overall responsibility for it.

The trial used 60 New Zealand white/Lop cross rabbits aged 16–24 weeks, split into 10 groups, each with a different diet. Four of the groups were given A1 beta-casein in amounts varying up to 20% of the diet, and four were given A2 beta-casein. Two groups received whey protein that contained neither A1 nor A2 beta-casein. Some groups also received additional cholesterol, which was known to induce fatty plaques in the arteries of this breed of rabbits.

Each rabbit had its right carotid artery 'balloon de-endotheliased' prior to the trial. This is a surgical procedure commonly used in trials of this kind, to make the rabbits more prone to atherosclerosis. The endothelium is a single layer of cells lining the inside of arteries, and damage to it is believed to play an important (but not fully understood) role in causing atherosclerosis. The damage may increase the chance of fatty plaques being laid down in a reasonably short time. As long as all animals in the trial are treated the same way this procedure introduces no bias when comparing one treatment with another.

Prior to this trial it had already been widely reported in the scientific literature that casein was linked to atherosclerosis, and Campbell's team referred to previous research that found this with rabbits, monkeys and mice. However, none of these previous studies had looked at which particular component of casein, if any, was the problem.

What they found was that rabbits fed A1 beta-casein developed fatty plaque lesions that were both larger and thicker than those of rabbits fed A2 beta-casein. Interestingly, and perhaps surprisingly, the biggest differences were in the undamaged aorta (the main artery that exits from the heart) rather than in the damaged carotid artery. The differences in relation to the aorta were statistically significant, some at the $p< 0.05$ level and others at the $p< 0.01$ level, which indicates that the probability of getting these differences by chance is less than 5% and 1%, respectively. The team said that the lesions that were formed 'are termed fatty streaks and closely resemble juvenile fatty streaks that are present in early childhood and are considered the precursors of advanced atherosclerotic plaques'. They concluded that their results 'demonstrate for the first time that beta-casein A2 has a mildly athero-protective effect while beta-casein A1 is most definitely atherogenic'.

Campbell and her team also found some evidence, although only in groups that had no added dietary cholesterol, that the rabbits on A2 diets had lower serum cholesterol levels than those fed A1. They suggested that any effects in the groups fed additional cholesterol might have been masked by these dietary supplements. However, it is debatable whether the higher serum cholesterol levels with A1 beta-casein have much meaning. There is no obvious mechanism whereby BCM7 from A1 beta-casein would have a primary effect on serum cholesterol levels, whereas there is a mechanism whereby the fatty plaques might be laid down. (I will discuss this later in this chapter.) But the results were statistically significant, so they cannot be ignored. It may well be that the cholesterol effect was a secondary effect.

Not surprisingly, publication of this paper brought the A1 and A2 protagonists out of their corners. One of the more interesting responses was from Professor Sir John Scott, a retired eminent cardiologist and former President of the Royal Society of New Zealand (the foremost science body, to which most New Zealand scientists belong, and which has nothing to do with royalty). Professor Scott appears not to have previously taken a public position in relation to A2 milk, but he was interviewed in 2003 for the Four Corners programme 'White Mischief'. He emphasised the importance of Campbell's work, saying that the trials 'were extremely well done, because she has such a justified high reputation of research and because the results were so clear-cut ... it's an ostrich attitude not to accept that and act accordingly.'[1]

Some others were not so sure. The paper first became available online in about May 2003. (Many journals now make a paper available to subscribers through the internet as soon as it has been accepted for publication and processed through to the final proofs. At this stage it has been peer-reviewed and is deemed to be of an acceptable scientific standard. Typically a few months then go by before the print version is available.) In this case the print version of the journal was dated September, and included an editorial by Professors Jim Mann and Murray Skeaff from Otago University, attacking the Campbell paper. They also took the opportunity to have a go at the epidemiology, but I will focus here on the specifics of the Campbell paper.

Essentially, their argument was that there is a huge leap from the results of one trial with rabbits to the claims made by Campbell and her team. Mann and Skeaff pointed out that the rabbits in this trial got artery thickening in the aorta (the main artery emerging from the heart), whereas in humans thickening typically occurs in the coronary, carotid and femoral arteries. Also, they argued there was a huge difference between animals developing arterial plaque in a period of months, and humans developing it over a period of years.

So how should we interpret this and how much weight should we put on the rabbit trial? The points made by Mann and Skeaff are correct in a technical sense. If this were the only evidence then by itself it would be insufficient to prove that A1 beta-casein caused heart disease in humans. But in terms of the overall jigsaw puzzle of A1 milk, the results with rabbits are surely very important. Professor Campbell's work tells us that at least in one species of animal there is very strong evidence that A1 beta-casein induces heart disease whereas A2 beta-casein does not, and that the signs of this become evident and statistically convincing after only six weeks on the different diets.

Mice: flawed research

There is one other animal trial of interest and this was led by Dr Greg Dusting at the Howard Florey Institute in Melbourne. This research used what are called 'ApoE mice', which have a genetic deficiency in the ApoE gene. As a consequence, the blood of these mice lacks apolipoprotein – a factor which is essential for carrying cholesterol to and from the arterial tissues. The ApoE gene is also very important in humans, and people with a deficient ApoE gene are susceptible to a range of conditions including heart disease and Alzheimer's disease. According to Dusting's comments on the Four Corners programme in 2003, ApoE mice that had received the A2 diet had a slightly higher area of lesions than those that had received the A1 diet. The phrase 'slightly higher' probably means that the differences were not statistically significant and therefore there is no confidence that a repeat trial would find any difference. Unfortunately this work has never been published and presumably it never will, as the trials were undertaken more than four years ago. Were ApoE mice a good choice of animal for this work? Perhaps not, as it meant inevitably that their blood would be overloaded with cholesterol regardless of the treatment to which they were subjected. Also, as Julie Campbell pointed out, whereas rabbits carry their cholesterol in a very similar way to the way humans do, 'rats and mice carry their cholesterol completely differently.'[2]

Unfortunately there are no answers to these questions. It is impossible to place weight on a trial that has never been published. It is a fairly sure sign when this happens that some aspect of the trial was sufficiently flawed that the scientists know that they won't get ready acceptance by the peer reviewers. Dr Andrew Clarke, who was Chief Executive Officer of A2 Corporation, has suggested to me that this trial actually supports the A2 hypothesis, in that these specially bred mice did not have a crucial component of the biological mechanism by which A1 beta-casein damages the heart. Hence we would not expect A1 beta-casein to act any differently than A2 beta-casein in these mice.

So why have I devoted space to describing a trial that told us nothing? For the simple reason that this unpublished and apparently flawed trial is one of the pieces of so-called 'evidence' that detractors use to discredit the A2 hypothesis. Indeed Fonterra's Jeremy Hill has, in correspondence to me, been critical of A2 Corporation for not publishing this work. But it is not incumbent upon A2 Corporation to publish this work. They were only the people who funded it. Publication was the task of the scientists who did the investigations. Dr Clarke has advised me in writing that there are no restraints imposed by his company on the publication of this work. He has also supplied me with the unpublished report supplied to A2 Corporation by the scientists. But of course if publication were to occur then these independent scientists who did the work would have to get it accepted by a journal and its peer reviewers.

Scientific mechanisms

If A1 beta-casein and hence BCM7 have an effect on human heart disease there must be a biological mechanism that is making this happen. In this section I will look at what that mechanism might be.

The immediate assumption of many people is that it will be cholesterol related. However, the chances of this being the primary mechanism are slim. Quite simply, the difference between A1 and A2 beta-casein has no obvious direct link with serum cholesterol. If there is a cholesterol link then it is likely to be a secondary effect, i.e. whatever is causing the heart disease also affects serum cholesterol. Or perhaps there is no real effect at all. Nevertheless, Julie Campbell's rabbit work did indicate that there might be some sort of a link, so it was important that this should be investigated.

A group at Otago University, including Professors Jim Mann and Murray Skeaff who wrote the *Atherosclerosis* editorial about Julie Campbell's work, decided to do just that. They compared the blood cholesterol levels in adults who were placed on a diet where their dairy consumption came either from ordinary milk (containing a mixture of A1 and A2 beta-caseins) or from specialist A2 milk. Their work was first published online in *Atherosclerosis* in November 2005.

Half of the participants were put on an ordinary-milk diet for four weeks and then spent four weeks on an A2 diet. The other participants spent the first four weeks on A2 milk and then changed to A1. None of the participants knew which type of milk they were consuming at any particular time.

The results showed no difference between the two types of milk in regard to total cholesterol, LDL cholesterol ('bad' cholesterol), HDL cholesterol ('good' cholesterol) or triacylglycerol.[3] Regardless of diet, total cholesterol, LDL cholesterol and triacylglycerol dropped compared to the figures at the start. The participants were on average consuming about 34 grams of cheese and just under 0.5 litres of milk per day. So it seems fairly clear that the A1 and A2 beta-caseins have no effect on cholesterol, at least in the short term and with this level of intake. So we indeed have to look elsewhere for a mechanism.

The Otago University results came as no surprise to me. In fact when the trial was being set up I wrote to Jim Mann urging him and his colleagues to take additional measurements, including BCM7 in blood and urine, and an LDL oxidation assay. The response came from Murray Skeaff. We had an email correspondence that started off on very friendly terms but subsequently came to an abrupt end.

Skeaff's first response included the following:

> It is possible to test the cholesterolaemic effects of A1 vs A2 beta-casein protein in a trial with human participants and this is what we are doing. Our study is by no means a definitive study to test all of the potential differential effects of A1 and A2 casein on physiological and metabolic events linked with atherogenesis. We have a very small budget for the project and are doing what we can. Do you have some funds that could be used to fund some additional measurements?

I responded that I did not have access to funds, but offered to help them as follows:

> Presumably the only people likely to fund a project like this would be Fonterra or A2 Corporation. I am sure that I have no influence with Fonterra on matters such as this, at least in the short term. I

would have to work the long way via some directors whom I know rather than through management. I presume you have already talked to Fonterra about this?

In the case of A2 Corporation I would be happy to talk with Andrew Clarke. Andrew and I have never met in person but we do correspond electronically, and occasionally by telephone. I think I have a fair idea as to his thinking.

My guess is that A2 would be very interested in seeing that some other measurements were undertaken, and they may be prepared to fund if they were happy with the protocol. In saying this I am aware that there has been some tension between your group and A2 in the past. It would be a pity if that were to get in the way, and I would be happy to talk to Andrew about this.

In the absence of immediate funding would it be possible to take bloods and freeze them for later analysis? Presumably you will already be planning to take bloods at the start, end, and also at diet crossover time? Do you have a rough idea as to the additional funds that would be required?

Murray Skeaff responded: 'Thank-you for your offer to help obtain funds but we have intentionally stayed away from soliciting funds from any company with an interest in A1 or A2.' He also added: 'LDL-oxidation measurement, which we have done in other work, requires immediate ultracentrifugation of blood samples once collected. This is time consuming and beyond the resources of our study.'

I thought it was a huge pity that they didn't take these additional measurements. The trial was actually quite expensive: the milk products alone for 62 people for eight weeks would have cost over NZ$5000. Then there was all the time of the investigators, plus the unpaid contributions of the participants. It is no big deal to ultracentrifuge blood samples: I know that from other work I have been involved in with animals.

In fact I was quite irritated by the design of this trial. A couple of months after our email conversations, but well before there was any indication of what the Otago team had found, I wrote the following as part of a long article aimed at farm consultants (who advise farmers on issues such as breeding strategy), in the journal *Primary Industry Management*:[4]

There has been a recent trial at University of Otago testing the effect of

> A1 and A2 milk on cholesterol levels, for which the results are forthcoming. But I doubt if it will prove much. Testing the A2 hypothesis requires testing for BCM7 in the bloodstream and urine, and also testing for LDL oxidation. Whether or not there will be a differential effect on cholesterol is doubtful, and my best guess based on what is already known about casein is that they may find that both the A1 and A2 diets lead to a reduction in blood cholesterols over the period of the trial. I have tried to convince the researchers involved to take blood samples, centrifuge the contents, and then store on ice for subsequent detailed analysis when funds are available. But alas, it is not happening.

Murray Skeaff subsequently took me to task by email for making those comments, but they were absolutely true, not only in relation to my communication with the researchers, but in my predictions of the outcomes. The results showed no difference in cholesterol levels between the A1 and A2 diets, and they did show, for both treatments, a reduction in blood cholesterols over the period of the trial. It was exactly what I had predicted!

Actually the reason I expected this reduction had nothing to do with the casein itself. When people join a trial such as this it tends to make them think more about health issues. Either consciously or subconsciously they therefore take more care over the food they eat. Hence, regardless of which trial diet they were on, there was a likelihood that the participants' cholesterol levels would drop.

My irritation was increased by a press release from the Otago team while the trial was being set up, in which one of the researchers reportedly said that the purpose was to prove or disprove the A2 hypothesis. Clearly no such proof either way could be established unless a lot more relevant measurements were taken and analysed, such as LDL oxidation and BCM7 in blood and urine – a point that Murray Skeaff later conceded in an email. However, my ire was further raised when the paper was published in *Atherosclerosis* and the authors did indeed go beyond their data to speculate on LDL-oxidation-related issues:

> Another mechanism by which beta-casein has been suggested to be atherogenic is by the release of a peptide (BCM7) in the small intestine, its presumed passage into blood, and its presumed ability to oxidize LDL. However, BCM7 is released by both the A1 and B

> variants, and a slightly longer peptide, BCM9, is released from the A2 variant of beta-casein. It is difficult to reconcile how these two similar peptides, BCM7 and BCM9, might exert biological effects that differ to the extent that one is supposed to be atherogenic whilst the other is not.

However, there are at least three reasons why we know that BCM9 is quite different to BCM7. First, it is a bigger molecule than BCM7 so it can't enter the bloodstream so easily. To the best of my knowledge no-one has ever measured BCM9 as getting through into the blood or urine. Secondly, work by Japanese scientists Yunden Jinsmaa and Masa-aki Yoshikawa (whom the Otago team reference in their own work) has shown that BCM9 not only generates lower opioid activity than BCM7, but also has only about one-quarter the binding affinity to opioid receptors that BCM7 has.[5] So, to use an analogy, we know that BCM7 has more horsepower and more torque than BCM9, and that it can also get through tunnels in which BCM9 gets stuck. There are lots of things we still have to learn about both BCM7 and BCM9, but we certainly know that they are quite different.

And just to complicate the story a little more, there are at least three versions of BCM9, all with different properties. Not only is there human BCM9 and bovine BCM9 from A1 beta-casein, which differ in three out of nine amino acids and have quite different properties, but there is also a bovine BCM9 from A2 beta-casein. The BCM9 from A1 beta-casein has a histidine in the eighth position, where the BCM9 from A2 beta-casein has a proline. Jinsmaa and Yoshikawa have shown that this apparently subtle difference has a big impact on both the 'horsepower' and the 'torque'.

One of my frustrations with trying to work through the issues of BCM7 is that many people have a pre-existing stance. All of us have difficulty in reversing a pre-existing position we have taken on an issue. And most people in a debate are quick to see the evidence that supports their position and to downplay the evidence that is contrary to it. This seems to be human nature. As the Scottish author and poet Andrew Lang put it, people often use statistics the way a drunk man uses a lamp-post: for support rather than illumination. And when the arguments depend on the complexities of biochemistry and pharmacology, it is very easy for the light on the lamp-post to be obscured by fog.

There is another trial looking at cholesterol effects, published in 2006 but actually undertaken several years earlier, by an Australian group with Jaye Chin-Dusting as the lead author. They obtained similar results to the Otago group. They used higher intakes of casein than the Otago group but only had six men and nine women in their study. They too found no effect on cholesterol. But unfortunately their trial was confounded because the so-called 'A2 diet' contained up to 20% A1!

The Otago group also reported A1 contamination in their A2 milk. I took this up with Dr Andrew Clarke, the CEO of A2 Corporation. The issue was important not only in relation to the trial but also because the Otago group had obtained their A2 milk from commercial sources. Was this commercial A2 milk really a mix of A1 and A2 milk? Clarke was quick to respond, and sent me lots of laboratory test results undertaken by Food Science Australia and also by Mimonics Pty Ltd, a company that specialises in mass-spectral analyses. These results showed how the particular methods used by the Otago team, based on non-calibrated capillary electrophoresis (CE), always show apparent contamination even when it does not exist. In other words, the contamination in the Chin-Dusting trial was real (measured using appropriate techniques), but that in the Otago trial was not. If nothing else, this shows how complex and confusing the path of science can be. I have more to say about these inaccurate CE tests in Chapter 11.

So if cholesterol is not a key component of the biological pathway then what can this pathway be? There are two promising possibilities, or perhaps it is a combination of the two possibilities working together. We know for sure that BCM7 is a powerful opioid. And we also know for sure that BCM7 is a powerful oxidant. The term 'oxidant' is widely used in health articles but what does it really mean?

Originally oxidation meant the addition of oxygen, but nowadays it more generally means any reaction that involves the loss of an electron. An oxidant is therefore a molecule that removes an electron from another molecule. This can create what is called a free radical, which then sets up a chain reaction whereby other molecules are oxidised. When LDL (the 'bad' cholesterol) is oxidised it tends to stick to the arteries and form fatty plaque. The oxidised LDL may also cause the artery wall to become inflamed and this may make it more sticky.

The oxidation and hence plaque-forming process is stopped by antioxidants. According to the theory, if we consume lots of antioxidants, which tend to stop these reactions from occurring, and minimise our intake of oxidants, then our chances of getting atherosclerosis and having a heart attack are reduced. The best way to consume lots of antioxidants is to eat plenty of fruit and vegetables.

As with so many issues relating to human health there remains a huge amount that we do not know. But we do know that oxidised LDL is a major cause for concern. And we also know on theoretical grounds that BCM7, with its tyrosine amino acid at one end plus its high resistance to breakdown, will be a powerful oxidant. In fact French scientists Jean Torreilles and Marie-Christian Guerin have shown that BCM7 does indeed oxidise LDL.[6] Also, Czech scientist A. Steinerova and colleagues have published several papers showing that infants exposed to cows' milk have up to ten times more antibodies to oxidised LDL than babies that are breastfed.[7] Steinerova and colleagues have postulated that this is caused by A1 beta-casein. So this is an evolving story, with quite a lot known but still much more to be discovered.

There is another slant to the mechanism story which I have yet to mention, apart from a passing reference in Chapter 1 to the Sippy diet. Dr Sippy was an American physician who lived in the late 19th and early 20th century. According to *Dorland's Medical Dictionary* (online) the Sippy diet is 'a diet formerly used to treat peptic ulcers, consisting of milk, cream and other supposedly bland foods; it was later proved ineffective.'

Not only was this diet ineffective: it was subsequently found to cause high rate of death from heart attacks. The key paper is by R.D. Briggs and four co-authors and was published in 1960 in the medical journal *Circulation*.[8] They undertook an autopsy study in 15 hospitals in the USA and Great Britain. In Great Britain they found that the death rate from myocardial infarction (heart attacks) amongst ulcer sufferers was nearly 2.5 times as high among those on the Sippy and other high-milk diets compared to those not on a milk diet. In the USA the heart attack death rate of ulcer sufferers on the Sippy diet was six times that of ulcer sufferers not on the Sippy diet. In both countries the results were highly significant, at $p < 0.01$. When taken together, this means that the likelihood of getting two sets of results like this from a random effect or 'fluke' (i.e. a false association) is less than one in ten thousand. So we can be very confident this is a real effect involving causation linked to milk intake. And the medical profession did indeed respond to these results: the Sippy diet rapidly fell out of favour in the 1960s. At the time it was thought the problem probably related to the high fat intake on this diet. In those days nothing at all was known about the beta-caseins.

What we now understand is that people with stomach ulcers have a damaged digestive system so it is much easier for peptides (protein fragments) as well as single amino acids to get into the bloodstream. People with ulcers are just one part of a much bigger group who for various reasons suffer from a leaky gut, more formally described as 'enhanced digestive permeability'. It is this leaky gut that allows the BCM7 to sneak into the bloodstream and then to do its damage in a multiplicity of ways. It seems likely that the particular damage it does depends on the genetic makeup of the person, and for many people it is the cardiovascular system that suffers damage. So probably not all of us are at risk of heart disease from A1 beta-casein and BCM7. It is only going to be those people who for one reason or another have a leaky gut.

I will talk a lot more about leaky gut syndrome, as it is a key issue that seems to unify all the disease conditions with which BCM7 is associated. Unfortunately, for one reason or another a considerable number of people suffer from it. I regard the Briggs paper as being a very important piece of the jigsaw puzzle, although Briggs and his colleagues had no idea as to how and where it fitted.

The big picture

Having now heard about the epidemiology, the animal trials and the biochemistry, readers can make their own judgement as to whether they believe there is a link between A1 beta-casein, BCM7 and heart disease.

The most weighty argument against the heart-disease link is that no-one has ever proven in a double-blind trial that humans fed A1 beta-casein get more heart disease than those fed A2 beta-casein. (The principles of scientific investigation, including double blinding of both participants and investigators, are discussed in Appendix 1.) This is indeed true. Rather, it is a case of lots of individual pieces of a jigsaw puzzle. But if double-blind clinical trials were really the only acceptable evidence that justified action, we would still all be denying that smoking is harmful. This is because there has *never* been a double-blind trial of smoking and cancer. And there are some very obvious reasons why they would be impossible to conduct. It is much the same for A1 beta-casein and heart disease.

The question then becomes: how can we find that extra bit of proof that some people are going to demand before being convinced?

Proof is unlikely to come from epidemiology. The existing epidemiological evidence based on between-country analyses is already extremely strong and there is really nothing more to add. And in any case, one of the standard arguments of the doubters is that epidemiology can never prove anything.

Chances are that the inter-country epidemiology will if anything become less clear over time because of the effects of three different classes of drugs that are increasingly being used in the battle against heart disease. These are the statins (which reduce cholesterol and also act as anti-inflammatories on the artery walls), the good old aspirin and related drugs that thin the blood, and the ACE inhibitors (which make the arteries more pliant and less likely to get clogged). Because these drugs have been introduced at different times in different countries they will tend to confound the previously simple story.

Nor will the doubters be convinced by more animal trials. Another of their standard claims is that such trials can never prove anything in regard to humans. It would be nice to see a repeat of Professor Julie Campbell's trials, perhaps with bigger numbers of rabbits and without cholesterol-enhanced diets, but that won't provide any great breakthroughs: the Campbell results are already very strong at a level that statisticians usually regard as being 'proof'.

Definitive human trials are also going to be difficult because heart disease in humans takes so long to develop. If I were designing human trials, I would focus on first identifying groups of people who for one reason or another were believed to have leaky guts, and testing their blood and urine for the presence of BCM7. And I would be checking their heart-disease mortality data.

And then there is the precautionary principle, according to which we should weigh up the cost of getting it wrong. What damage may we be doing by ignoring the evidence in relation to A1 beta-casein, if it turns out that BCM7 really is the milk devil? How does this potential cost compare with the monetary cost to farmers of shifting to A2 milk and later finding that it wasn't necessary after all? I will explore this monetary cost further in Chapter 10.

The links between A1 beta-casein and heart disease discussed in this chapter are of course only part of the BCM7 story, for there is evidence that the milk devil has many more tricks to play. It is therefore now time to look at diabetes, and then autism, schizophrenia and many other auto-immune diseases.

NOTES

1 Australian Broadcasting Corporation 2003. *White Mischief.* Available at www.abc.net.au/4corners/content/2003/transcripts/s820943.htm

2 *New Zealand Herald*, 7 April 2003.

3 Triacylglycerol is also commonly referred to as 'triglyceride'.

4 See Woodford (2004a) in Industry, Marketing and Overview section of Bibliography.

5 See Jinsmaa and Yoshikawa (1999) in Milk and Casomorphins section of Bibliography.

6 See Toreilles and Guerin (1995) in Heart Disease section of Bibliography.

7 See papers by Steinerova in Heart Disease section of Bibliography.

8 See Briggs *et al* (1950) in Heart Disease section of Bibliography.

CHAPTER FIVE

POPULATION EVIDENCE FOR TYPE 1 DIABETES

As with heart disease, there are several parts to the diabetes story. The first part, relating to epidemiology, is told in this chapter. It shows that the incidence of Type 1 diabetes is much higher in countries where there is a high intake of A1 beta-casein, than in countries where the intake is lower. The second part, about animal trials, is in Chapter 6. The third part, about what has been found in humans and how the different parts of the diabetes jigsaw puzzle fit together, is covered in Chapter 7.

As with all chapters of this book, this one is not just about science but also about how people choose to present that science. The diabetes story is full of human intrigue. It is a battle between competing individuals and organisations. Big dollars, big egos and research grants are all at stake.

The A2 story actually began with diabetes. Then, as the years went by, the heart-disease investigations and the diabetes investigations developed together, at times in parallel and at other times with one field of investigation surging ahead of the other. I chose to tell the heart-disease story first (Chapters 3 and 4), but I could just as easily have chosen the diabetes story.

The story of how Professor Bob Elliott began researching A1 beta-casein as a possible cause of Type 1 diabetes has already been introduced in Chapter 1. It was an inspired combination of intuition and deduction by Bob Elliott and Jeremy Hill that set things in motion back in 1993. Without their complementary talents and knowledge, the milk devil might have remained unknown for a lot longer.

Many people get confused between the two types of diabetes, so I will start with a reminder of the distinction. Type 1 diabetes typically (but not always) develops in childhood or young adulthood and at present has no cure. Type 1 diabetics suffer from a condition where their own body destroys the insulin-producing cells in the pancreas, so they require insulin injections every day for the rest of their lives. They also have increased risk factors for many other diseases including heart disease. In contrast, Type 2 diabetes typically develops later in life and hence is sometimes called late-onset diabetes. Most Type 2 diabetics do not require insulin injections. In fact Type 2 diabetes is not caused so much by a lack of insulin as by the body's resistance to allowing the insulin to transport the glucose into individual cells. There is very clear evidence that Type 2 diabetes is related to a range of lifestyle factors, and that people who exercise a lot and control their diet are unlikely to suffer from it.

Type 1 diabetes is one of many auto-immune diseases, i.e. where the body attacks itself. Other auto-immune diseases include multiple sclerosis, eczema, Parkinson's disease, coeliac disease and Crohn's disease. I am very suspicious about A1 beta-casein being a risk factor in relation to many of these diseases, either by being a direct link in the causation process or else by these diseases creating new opportunities for BCM7 to cross into the blood, but that is a story that can wait until Chapter 9.

In the case of Type 1 diabetes, without the insulin-producing cells in the pancreas, the body cannot metabolise sugars. Regular insulin injections provide nowhere near the level of sugar regulation in the blood that occurs with a properly functioning pancreas. Before insulin injections were available, Type 1 diabetics died at an early age. Even now they have many lifestyle restrictions, including being very careful about what they eat. They also have to monitor their blood sugar closely or else they set themselves up for a range of other health conditions. In the future, there may well be sophisticated genetic treatments based on stem-cell technology or other types of implanted cells that will make life easier for Type 1 diabetics. Those treatments, if they ever work, are still some time away. In fact Professor Bob Elliott is also one of the leading scientists working on implanting cells from pigs as a cure. He is having some success. But it would all be so much simpler if we could identify the factors that cause diabetes in the first place. Meanwhile, the worldwide incidence of Type 1 diabetes keeps increasing at about 3% a year.[1] About 65,000 children aged up to 14 are newly diagnosed each year[2] and there are almost as many additional new cases each year among young adults. The vast majority are in the developed world.

Scientists agree that some human genetic profiles (genotypes) are more susceptible to Type 1 diabetes than are others. The genetic variations that seem to be implicated are found in all races, although not necessarily in the same frequency. But it is very clear that genes are just part of the story. Having a particular gene, or variant of a gene (allele), only increases or decreases susceptibility. Even with identical twins it is common for one twin to become diabetic and the other to remain free of the disease. Accordingly, it seems very clear that some thing or things in the environment cause some people's auto-immune systems to go on the attack.

If there were a simple cause of Type 1 diabetes then science would have found that cause a long time ago. In all probability there is a range of risk factors. In some people with genetic susceptibility it might require only one environmental factor. In others it may require a combination of factors. Among possible triggers, viruses and diet are the prime candidates, acting either alone or together.[3]

The first peer-reviewed paper to be published on the epidemiology of diabetes and A1 beta-casein was authored by Bob Elliott (The University of Auckland), Jeremy Hill (NZDRI) and three colleagues, and published in 1999 in *Diabetologia*.[4]

Elliott and his team compared the incidence of diabetes in children aged 0–14 years with the intake of dairy protein, and in particular A1 beta-casein, in 10 countries – Australia, Canada, Denmark, Finland, Germany, Iceland, New Zealand, Norway, Sweden and the USA. The data for the USA came from the city of San Diego. A key feature of all these countries is that they are high-income western countries with a European-type lifestyle. This commonality is important because it reduces the likelihood of confounding factors.

Elliott and his team concluded that 'Total [milk] protein consumption did not correlate with diabetes incidence [r^2 =+0.16] but consumption of the beta-casein A1 variant did [r^2 = +0.53]. Even more pronounced was the relation between beta-casein (A1 + B) consumption and diabetes [r^2 = +0.96].'[5]

Two explanatory points may be helpful to the interpretation of this information. The first is a reminder that there are actually several variants of the beta-casein gene. In this book (and also commonly in the scientific journals) all variants with histidine at position 67 are lumped together and referred to as A1. All these variants can be expected to release BCM7 on digestion. Similarly, all variants that have proline at position 67 are referred to as A2. This is just a convenient shorthand, given that A1 and A2 are by far the most common variants. However, in their paper Bob Elliott and colleagues separated out the A1 and B variants in some of their analyses. What they call (A1+B) is therefore their way of saying the two most important variants that have histidine at position 67.

The second point is a reminder as to the interpretation of the r^2 values. These values tell us the proportion of the variation in the between-country disease incidence levels that can be explained by the intake of total milk protein and A1 beta-casein. Statistical tests can then be undertaken which measure whether the relationships are likely to be 'real' relationships or simply due to chance. In this case, the tests showed that the weak relationship between total milk protein and diabetes incidence was non-significant. In contrast, the relationships between the A1 beta-casein intake and diabetes, and the combined A1 + B beta-casein intake, are clearly significant from a statistical perspective. In the case of the A1 variant considered by itself, the statistical analysis showed that the probability of getting such a relationship through chance factors that have no real meaning is less than one in fifty ($p < 0.02$). In the case of the A1 and B variants considered together, the probability of getting such a relationship due to chance would be less than one in ten thousand ($p < 0.0001$).[6] *So it seems that Bob Elliott and colleagues were really onto something big. We can be very confident that, unless there is a third factor that affects both diabetes incidence and intake of A1 beta-casein, we do have a genuine relationship.*

One of the stand-out features of the data presented by Elliott and colleagues was that Iceland had the highest milk intake but quite moderate levels of Type 1 diabetes. This seemed to make sense because the Icelandic milk was indeed very low in A1 beta-casein (because of the predominance of the Norske breed). However, it seemed important to see whether there was anything else in the Icelandic milk that might be causing the low level of Type 1 diabetes relative to the nearby Nordic countries of Finland, Sweden, Norway and Denmark. Accordingly, a related group of workers took up this issue: two Icelanders (B. Birgisdottir and I. Thorsdottir) from the Unit for Nutrition Research at Landspitali-University Hospital, Iceland, and Jeremy Hill and D. Harris from the NZDRI.[7] Specifically, they looked at the levels of bovine serum albumin (BSA), immunoglobulin and lactoferrin. BSA was already suspected of causing diabetes and the others had been suggested elsewhere in the scientific literature as being potentially protective against diabetes. However, the researchers were unable to find any statistical relationship consistent with any of these hypotheses. In fact, for BSA they found that Icelanders had a higher intake than people in the other Nordic countries, so clearly this could not be the predominant cause of diabetes. They also concluded that the lower diabetes incidence in Iceland could not be ascribed to differences in breastfeeding habits, climate or infectious diseases. So although this study did nothing to further prove the A1 relationship with Type 1 diabetes, it did seem to disprove a number of alternative possibilities. It left the 'cupboard bare' in terms of suggestions as to what else could be the cause apart from A1 beta-casein and other A1-like variants of beta-casein.

Corran McLachlan, in his 2001 *Medical Hypotheses* paper, included some epidemiological data for diabetes but they were only a very minor part. His major interest was heart disease. For diabetes he found a high correlation ($r^2 = 0.75$). He obtained similar results both with cheese included and excluded, but obtained a poorer fit when the A1 variant and the B variant were added together. Unfortunately he did not report the correlation coefficient for the combined A1 and B beta-casein variants. Given the overall lack of detail that he provides for diabetes, there is little point in spending time analysing his diabetes results. Really, they are no more than a footnote to the emerging story. Corran McLachlan's remarkable contribution was to identify the link between A1 beta-casein and heart disease. Also, he identified the remarkable inter-country correlation between heart disease and Type 1 diabetes. Others had more to say about the links between A1 beta-casein and diabetes.

The most important work on diabetes epidemiology is Laugesen and Elliott's 2003 paper in the *New Zealand Medical Journal*, which paid great attention to both heart disease and diabetes and provided a comprehensive and methodical analysis (see Chapter 3). The paper lays out every step of the analysis so that other scientists can check exactly the assumptions that have been made and the analyses that have been undertaken. This is the way good science should be done, although the paper itself is hardly bedside reading. Given the cryptic nature of the prose, a casual reading can easily lead to misinterpretations of some of the things they are saying.

Laugesen and Elliott were able to find 19 countries for which there were data available on the A1 versus A2 beta-casein levels in the milk, and for which diabetes incidences were also reliably known. The diabetes data came from the World Health Organisation Diabetes Monitoring (WHO DiaMond) Project, except for the data for Switzerland and

Iceland, which were surveyed by the EuroDiab Ace study group. Thirteen of the countries were in Europe and the others were Australia, Israel, Japan, New Zealand, the USA and Venezuela. The data were for people aged 0–14 years and for the years 1990–94.

The correlations were remarkable. Considering A1 beta-casein from all dairy products except cheese, and excluding the minor variant B which also has histidine at position 67, the relationship had an r^2 value of 0.84. In other words, 84% of the variation in diabetes incidence can be explained by variation in A1 beta-casein intake. The probability of such a relationship showing up in the data by chance, if there was no causal

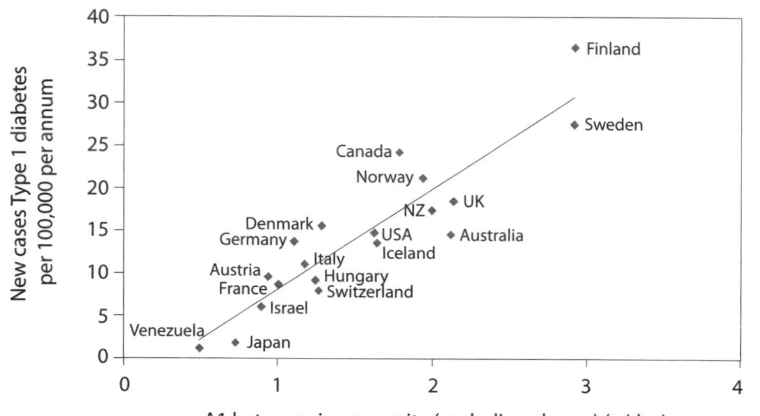

Fig. 5. Incidence of Type 1 diabetes and intake of A1 beta-casein excluding cheese.

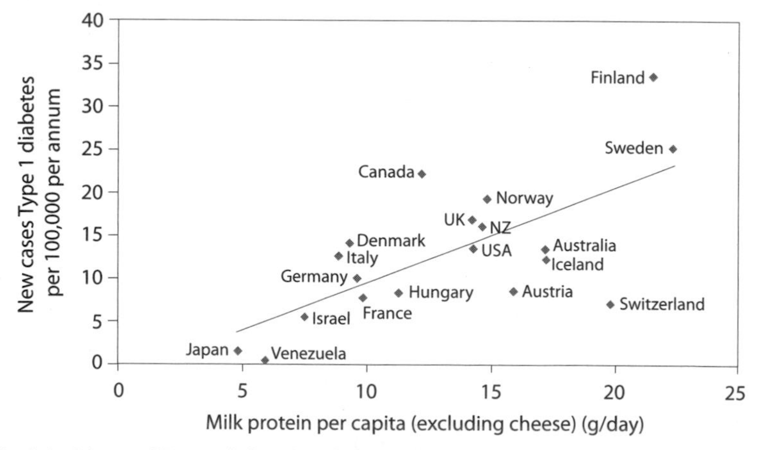

Fig. 6. Incidence of Type 1 diabetes and intake of milk protein excluding cheese.
(Data for both figures comes from Laugesen and Elliott (2003), *New Zealand Medical Journal* 116, (1168).)

relationship, is less than one in one thousand. Laugesen and Elliott were also able to show that although there was a positive relationship between diabetes incidence and total milk protein (also excluding cheese), the relationship was considerably weaker ($r^2 = 0.46$). (Figures 5 and 6).

Laugesen and Elliott also measured what is called the 'elasticity'. This measurement showed that a 1% decrease in the A1-like variants reduced the incidence of Type 1 diabetes by 1.3%. Once again, this is a very strong relationship.

They also looked at A1 beta-casein together with variant B. By doing so they got a somewhat lower r^2 of 0.74. There is no obvious reason why it should be lower, because there is no obvious reason why the variants that have histidine at position 67 should act differently to one another. It provides an interesting talking point, and it has been seized on by those who would like to discredit the epidemiology, but in all likelihood it is simply due to some random noise in the data. Statistically, the difference is not great enough to draw any conclusion in relation to the B variant (which is important only in a few countries) being different to A1.

Having said that there is no obvious reason why the B variant should act differently to A1, it would be wrong to totally exclude this possibility. Laugesen and Elliott stated that B beta-casein does have a different solubility and may be digested differently by the intestinal mucosa. In other words, the difference in the amino acid at position 122 that distinguishes A1 beta-casein from B beta-casein may cause the protein to fold differently and hence expose different parts of the molecule to digestive enzymes. But it may also simply be that the milk is pasteurised and processed differently (e.g. at different temperatures) in one country that happens to have higher levels of B beta-casein. Or it could be due to a small data error in the B variant in just one country. The correct statistical interpretation is that such small differences have no meaning. And the bottom line is that regardless of whether the B variant is included in the analysis, the relationship is amazingly strong.

What Laugesen and Elliott were also able to show was that there is a relationship between A2 beta-casein and incidence of diabetes ($r^2 = 0.22$), although this relationship was very much weaker than for A1 beta-casein, and also much weaker than for total protein. People who like to use statistics for support rather than illumination might therefore argue that A2 beta-casein is also implicated, but there is a much simpler explanation. Countries where people drink a lot of milk will tend to have a high intake of both A1 and A2 beta-casein. Hence, there is a level of what statisticians call co-linearity between these variables. In other words, there is a link between both A1 intake and A2 intake, and also between A1 intake and diabetes incidence. The A2 beta-casein is therefore being caught by this multiple association. There is no logical reason why this relationship (which is very much weaker than the correlation between A1 beta-casein and diabetes) should be regarded as causal. It is simply a case of the A2 beta-casein getting dragged along to a limited extent by the company that it has to keep. But it does provide some ammunition for those who would like to muddy the waters. And when dealing with statistics, and the low level of understanding that even many scientists have, it is easy for waters that should be crystal clear to become muddied!

Laugesen and Elliott also searched hard for relationships between diabetes and other foodstuffs. They also looked at non-food environmental factors. In all, they looked at over 170 foods and nutritional variables, but found few correlations. Diabetes tends to be more prevalent in northern European countries than in Mediterranean countries and hence there is an apparent correlation with both latitude and the northern European crops of oats and rye. But apparently there is no relationship between diabetes and the combined consumption of all the crops that contain gluten. (The reason why gluten might be important will become evident in Chapter 6.)

As for latitude, there are two possibilities. The first is that people in high-latitude countries receive less vitamin D from the sun. This has been identified as a possible risk factor for multiple sclerosis, and I will discuss this in Chapter 9, but it is not an obvious factor in Type 1 diabetes. The other possibility is that latitude is being dragged along by the company that it keeps. In general (and with the striking exception of Iceland), the northern European countries tend to be the high-A1 countries because of the predominant Holstein/Friesian, Ayrshire and Red Danish breeds, whereas in central and southern Europe the low-A1 breeds of Jersey, Simmental and Swiss Brown are more important.

Laugesen and Elliott made it clear that A1 and similar beta-casein variants were not the only risk factor for Type 1 diabetes. They pointed out that even in Guernsey, where there is minimal A1 beta-casein, there were five cases of Type 1 diabetes in the years 1990–1994, although the specifics of those cases have not been investigated (for example, did these people spend time elsewhere?) Also, Type 1 diabetes has been increasing steadily over recent decades despite there being a small decrease in the intake of A1 beta-casein. So something else is also a risk factor, perhaps interacting with the BCM7 from A1 beta-casein. I will leave that question until Chapter 7. But the big picture is very clear: *countries that have high A1 beta-casein intake have high incidence of Type 1 diabetes, and countries with low intake of A1 beta-casein have low incidence of diabetes.* And the statistical association is so strong that it cannot be classed as a fluke. It is a fact!

Whereas the counter-attack on the heart-disease epidemiology was quite strident, the Laugesen and Elliott epidemiological analyses of Type 1 diabetes have not been seriously criticised. However, Jeremy Hill, writing to the *New Zealand Medical Journal* from his position at that time of General Manager of the Fonterra Research Centre, claimed there were inconsistencies relative to other research.[8] He re-stated the issues about diabetes incidence increasing despite the decreasing consumption of A1 beta-casein. He also questioned why the inclusion of cheese weakened the relationship. But the answer to that is reasonably simple. First, it appears that the release of BCM7 from cheese is low (and possibly *very* low – see Chapter 2); and second, young children don't actually eat much cheese. Therefore, including cheese in the equations when it is mainly eaten by older groups in the population, could be expected to result in a confounding factor that would lower the correlations.

Another criticism from Hill related to the fact that inclusion of the B variant of beta-casein weakened the statistical relationships (although they were still very strong). This has already been discussed. And yet another comment related to the alleged importance of a paper investigating the relationship between A1 beta-casein and diabetes in rats and mice, that had been published a few months earlier. This study had been sponsored by the NZ Dairy Board (now part of Fonterra). I will be looking at this trial in great detail in the next chapter because of the non-disclosure of important information that was involved.

One of the fascinating issues is the way that Hill, previously co-author of at least three papers providing evidence in favour of the A2 hypothesis, was now taking the opposite position. The organisation that Hill worked for had also changed its stance. As pointed out in Chapter 1, in earlier times the NZDRI had applied for two patents, in one application arguing that A1 beta-casein was linked to diabetes, and in the other that it was linked to autism and schizophrenia. In those early days the New Zealand Livestock Improvement Corporation was also part of the New Zealand Dairy Board (as was the NZDRI). The issue was clearly considered important enough that someone put the word out to the Livestock Improvement Division that all bulls in the artificial-insemination programme should be tested for their A1 and A2 status. This testing programme has continued, and New Zealand is probably the only country in the world that knows the A1/A2 status of all its elite bulls.

Two other scientists who wrote to the *New Zealand Medical Journal* criticising the Laugesen and Elliott paper were Fraser Scott from the Ottawa Health Research Institute and Hubert Kolb from the German Diabetes Research Institute.[9] They too, like Jeremy Hill, were among the authors of the NZ Dairy Board-sponsored study involving rats and mice. And like Hill, they pointed out that their work with rats and mice did not support the Laugesen and Elliott stance in relation to A1 beta-casein as a risk factor. Well, we will soon see if that is the case, but first we need to look at some other types of epidemiology.

Diabetes and milk

The epidemiology I have been talking about so far has focused on A1 and A2 beta-casein. The only way to get these data has been to undertake comparisons between countries. But if such a relationship is real, and A1 beta-casein is an important risk factor for Type 1 diabetes, then within each country the children who drink a lot of milk will presumably be more likely to get diabetes than the children who don't. Also, the time when babies move from breastfeeding to either bovine milk or bovine-derived milk formulas might be important.

These within-country data are actually quite hard to get. Only a small proportion of children become diabetic and the disease may first manifest itself at different ages. It is difficult to collect food-intake data over long periods for large numbers of children. It is also difficult to get the parents of diabetic children to look back and accurately estimate their child's typical past daily intake of various foodstuffs. The way that a Finnish group led by Suvi Virtanen attacked these problems was to monitor the initially non-diabetic siblings of children who had developed diabetes.[10] They also undertook genetic testing of the children to identify which ones were more at risk. They then monitored these children using structured questionnaires for up to 11 years. Of the 725 children that they monitored, 33 developed diabetes.

They found that among these children (who because of the selection process tended to be genetically more susceptible than other children), those who drank more than three glasses (about 540 millilitres) of milk per day were more than five times more likely to become diabetic than those who drank less than three glasses per day. This result was statistically highly significant: the likelihood of getting it by chance was less than 1%. However, they were unable to find any statistically reliable relationship between the introduction non-human milk before or after two months of age and the subsequent rate of diabetes.

There have been a lot of other investigations of whether early introduction of bovine milk is a risk factor for Type 1 diabetes. Some studies have found such a relationship, but not all. A complicating factor is that some of the infant formula milks replace some or all of the casein protein with whey protein, and others do not. If the cause of the problem is A1 beta-casein, and hence BCM7, then whey-based formulas that exclude casein will not trigger diabetes. Paolo Pozzilli, a scientist from University Tor Vergata in Rome, concluded in a 1999 review that 'despite the conflicting data in this field, the underlying message is that exclusive breastfeeding for at least the first four months would be an easy way to reduce the risk of type 1 DM [diabetes mellitus] in children.'[11]

More recently B. Birgisdottir from Iceland and colleagues (including Jeremy Hill from Fonterra) have produced a further paper, published in the *Annals of Nutrition and Metabolism* in 2006, focusing specifically on the intake of A1 beta-casein of children aged 0–2 years, and also of adolescents aged 11–14. They found that it was in the 0–2 year age bracket where there was the greatest difference between Iceland and the Nordic countries (Norway, Sweden, Finland and Denmark) in intake of A1 beta-casein. Furthermore, the difference in diabetes incidence (number of new cases per year) between Iceland and these other countries was also greatest among young children aged 0–4 years.

They stated that their results supported the hypothesis that the crucial time in relation to exposure to A1 beta-casein was during early childhood.

Summary

As with heart disease, there is very strong evidence of a relationship between intake of A1 beta-casein and incidence of Type 1 diabetes. The relationships are so strong that it is highly unlikely that they could have occurred by chance. We do not have absolute proof of causation because epidemiology by itself can never provide absolute proof. But if there is no causation then what is the third factor that must be linked to both A1 beta-casein and the level of Type 1 diabetes? People such as Laugesen and Elliott have searched hard but without success for any such third factor that could explain this situation.

Using the same logic as for heart disease, it seems reasonable to at least consider the possibility that if A1 beta-casein causes Type 1 diabetes in humans then perhaps it might do something similar in at least some animal species. Also, it seems reasonable to hope that science would at least be able to provide some pointers to how this association might be occurring. These are the issues to be taken up in the next two chapters.

NOTES

1 See Onkamo *et al* (1999) in Diabetes section of Bibliography.

2 See the website of the International Diabetes Federation at www.eatlas.idf.org/Incidence/

3 There is strong evidence that the Coxsackie B4 virus can lead to auto-immune destruction of the pancreatic islet cells. But there appears to be no convincing evidence that this is a major cause of Type 1 diabetes. The Coxsackie family of enteroviruses are implicated in many health issues, including damage to the brain, heart (myocarditis), liver and skeletal system.

4 See Elliott *et al* (1999) in Diabetes section of Bibliography.

5 Laugesen and Elliott presented the correlation data as r, the correlation coefficient. I have converted these r values to r^2, which is known as the coefficient of determination. This conversion is in part for consistency of statistical presentation within this book and also because the coefficient of determination is easier to interpret.

6 These p-levels, also known as significance levels, are calculated in the statistical programmes which scientists use to analyse their results.

7 See Birgisdottir *et al* (2002) in Diabetes section of Bibliography.

8 See Hill (2003) in Diabetes section of Bibliography.

9 See Scott and Kolb (2003) in Diabetes section of Bibliography.

10 See Virtanen *et al* (2000) in Diabetes section of Bibliography.

11 See Pozzilli (1999) in Diabetes section of Bibliography.

CHAPTER 6

DIABETIC RODENTS AND SCIENTIFIC DISCLOSURE

Two types of rodent are widely used to study Type 1 diabetes. One is the non-obese diabetic mouse, usually referred to as the NOD mouse. The other is the BioBreeding rat (BB rat), named after the laboratory in Ottawa where it was originally bred. Both these specially-bred types spontaneously develop high rates of diabetes, the incidence varying depending on the particular colony and the nature of the diet. Bob Elliott has worked with these rodents for more than 20 years. As far back as 1984, in a paper published in *Diabetologia*, he showed that gluten (from cereals such as wheat, barley and rye) and casein were two proteins implicated in causing diabetes in the BB rat.[1] He was also able to demonstrate that whey protein (also from milk) was not diabetogenic. However, it was not until his momentous conversation with Jeremy Hill in 1993 that he thought to investigate whether there was any difference in diabetogenic (i.e. diabetes-inducing) effect between A1 and A2 beta-casein.

Bob Elliott and his team received funding from both the National Child Health Research Foundation and the New Zealand Dairy Board (now Fonterra) to undertake trials. The results they obtained, working with the NOD mouse, seemed to be very clear-cut. None of the mice fed the A2 beta-casein got diabetes but 47% of those fed A1 beta-casein did. Throughout the trial, some of the mice fed A1 beta-casein were also given the opioid-reversal drug naloxone in their drinking water. These mice also did not get diabetes. This seemed to say very clearly that the substance in milk that caused diabetes was BCM7, from A1 beta-casein, and that the effect was linked to its opioid (narcotic) characteristics.

There are two potential criticisms of these trials. The first is that the investigators were not ‘blind’ to which mice were getting which treatment. In medical science this is frowned upon as it creates opportunities for observational bias, whether conscious or unconscious. However, the biochemical tests for diabetes are very clear-cut and it should be impossible for accidental bias to intrude. (For example, if you dip a litmus paper into acid there is little likelihood that you will misread it as blue when it's red; but if you are observing rats that have fed on something you expect will make them sick you may be more likely to *think* they look sick. This is an example of the difference between objective and subjective observation. In Bob Elliott's trial the measurements were objective.)

The second criticism is that Bob Elliott and his colleagues published this work in a volume of conference proceedings,[2] which does not usually carry the same weight as publication in a peer-reviewed scientific journal. In fact the methods and the results, as set out in both the paper and the ensuing patent application,[3] are very impressive. It is disappointing that it was not published in a major international journal where more scientists could easily access the information.

The next step was to undertake a large-scale international trial using both BB rats and NOD mice. Where the initiative for this work came from is not clear, but it was sponsored by the NZ Dairy Board and involved animal-research laboratories in Great Britain, Canada and New Zealand. Scientists and technicians at the New Zealand Dairy Research Institute (also now part of Fonterra) were responsible for preparing the diets.

The paper reporting the trial was published in *Diabetologia* in 2002 and had nine co-authors.[4] This trial was called the Food and Diabetes (FAD) trial but the paper itself is sometimes referred to as the Beales *et al* paper because P.E. Beales from St Bartholomew's Hospital in London is the first listed author. However, it is Fraser Scott, at that time employed by the Ottawa Health Research Institute, who is listed as the corresponding author, which indicates it is he who stands first in line when it comes to explaining and defending what has been written. In fact all the authors except Fraser Scott (who is listed last) are listed in alphabetical order. In all, the nine authors list their national affiliations as the UK, Canada, New Zealand, Germany and Italy.

It was a complex trial with two species of rodents, three laboratories (each in a different country) and nine diets.

The first point to be clear on is that in each country only one type of rodent was used. In Britain they used a strain of mice known as NOD/

Ba (*NOD* = non-obese diabetogenic mice; *Ba* = St Bartholomew's Hospital). About 70% of these mice spontaneously develop diabetes by 30 weeks of age when fed a standard cereal-based laboratory feed. In New Zealand they used NOD/NZ mice which have about a 40% incidence of diabetes by 30 weeks of age. In Canada they used BB rats which exhibit a 60–70% incidence of diabetes at 30 weeks.

The second point to note is that the same suite of nine diets was used in all three countries. Four of the diets used a casein-based product called Pregestimil as the base and another four used a soy-based product called Prosobee. Both of these products are human infant formulas produced and marketed by Mead Johnson. To each of these base diets was then added either nothing, 10% whole casein, 10% A1 beta-casein or 10% A2 beta-casein. The ninth and last diet was a cereal-based milk-free rodent diet. One of the aims of putting together these different combinations was to produce some experimental diets that contained potential for the release of BCM7, and some that did not. All these diets were put together at the NZDRI and shipped to the different countries.

Third, it is important to remember that these rodents were all specially bred and selected to be susceptible to diabetes when fed a cereal-based diet. Even prior to the trial it was known that these particular genotypes were typically more susceptible to diabetes when fed cereal-based diets than when fed milk-based diets. So the real comparisons of interest were the direct comparisons between the A1 and A2 diets.

And that is what we are going to focus on in this chapter, at least initially. Once we apply our attention specifically to comparing A1 and A2 diets then everything becomes much more stark. This means just looking at A1 versus A2 beta-casein in rats in Canada, mice in England, and mice in New Zealand.

The first calamity to befall the trial was that the New Zealand mice suffered from an outbreak of *Clostridium* disease and many of them died. As a result, this part of the trial (under Bob Elliott's supervision) had to be abandoned. So now the trial was looking at just BB rats in Canada and NOD mice in England.

The second calamity was that the Pregestimil used as the base of some of the diet regimes already contained a 'high amount of BCM7', according to Jeremy Hill's document of October 2000. (This document was introduced in Chapter 1, and is reproduced in full as Appendix 2.) This meant that half the A2 diets were contaminated with BCM7, the nasty peptide released on digestion of A1 beta-casein. The comparison of A1 and A2 beta-casein within Pregestimil-based diets had therefore become a nonsense. It meant that this part of the trial was hopelessly confounded.

Amazingly, the paper published in *Diabetologia* makes no mention of this diet problem. Yet the paper was not submitted to the journal until 21 January 2002, with the final revised version received on 15 April 2002 and the paper finally published (initially online) on 19 July 2002. The submission date was well over a year after Jeremy Hill had told Warren Larsen that NZDRI had 'shown that Pregestimil contains a high amount of BCM7. This result is not known outside the NZ dairy industry and forms the basis of a confidential NZDRI Report.'

But the issue does not stop there. Jeremy Hill is actually *one of the authors* of the paper published in *Diabetologia*.

I believe this is a huge issue. The NZDRI was responsible for putting the diets together for the trial, but some time before October 2000 knew that it had supplied diets that were contaminated with BCM7. One of their scientists, who by his own words knew of the problem, then became a co-author of a scientific paper that made no mention of it.

If science is to progress then there has to be absolute disclosure in matters such as this. The FAD trial keeps being cited by those who disagree with the A2 hypothesis, without any mention of this confounding problem. This then misleads other scientists. Fraser Scott and Hubert Kolb themselves, as FAD-trial co-authors, referred to the trial in a letter to the *New Zealand Medical Journal* in March 2003, and used it as evidence against the A2 hypothesis in regard to diabetes.[5] Jeremy Hill and co-authors also referred to it in some of their papers at the 2003 International Dairy Federation Conference.[6] Stewart Truswell from Sydney University (who was also Fonterra's expert witness in the patent proceedings referred to in Chapters 3 and 11) has written in glowing terms about this paper in his own review in the *European Journal of Clinical Nutrition* in 2005.[7] He states (without any disclosure of his own links to Fonterra) that it is an 'important paper' and refers to its 'distinguished international panel of authors'.

Worse still, in 2006 in the same journal Truswell wrote in relation to this trial that 'any reader of the literature must surely take the findings of experienced researchers in Ottawa, London (England) and Auckland as the latest (perhaps the final) word on this subject.'[8]

And while this has been going on there has been no public acknowledgement from any of those involved that the diets were contaminated and that the trial was therefore confounded. Indeed the FAD trial was a total shambles.

So what were the supposed findings of the FAD trial as reported in *Diabetologia*? In essence they found that the cereal-based diet gave the highest rate of diabetes. This was not surprising. Given the way the rodents had been bred, it could have been predicted before the trial began. Apart from that, the message was not particularly clear. This has meant that the authors could assert both in that paper, and then more strongly when writing elsewhere, that the trial did not in general support the earlier findings of Bob Elliott's team, that A1 beta-casein was diabetogenic compared to A2 beta-casein. However, once the Pregestimil-treated animals for which there was major BCM7 contamination in the diets are excluded from the analysis, and we focus on the rodents fed Prosobee-based diets, with either A1 or A2 beta-casein added, then a somewhat different picture emerges. What we find is that the rats in Canada did indeed develop a much higher and statistically significant incidence of diabetes when fed A1 milk than when they were fed A2 milk (46% compared to 19%). (This result was recorded in the paper in the details of a table, but was not discussed.)

In contrast, in the case of the St Bartholomew's mice there was no significant difference, even with the Prosobee diets, between the animals fed A1 beta-casein and those fed A2 beta-casein. However, there is another analysis that we can do with the St Bartholomew's mice and that is to compare all of the animals fed Progestimil-based diets with those fed Prosobee-based diets. This shows an overall 41% incidence of diabetes in animals fed Pregestimil, compared to 31% for those fed Prosobee. And yet another insight from the trial is that animals fed whole casein (containing both A1 and A2 beta-casein) plus Prosobee developed a higher incidence of diabetes than those fed on Prosobee alone.

So the overall message from this trial, rather than what was concluded in *Diabetologia* and subsequently asserted elsewhere even more strongly by some of the authors, is now starting to look generally supportive of Elliott's earlier work. In summary, the Canadian rats had a much higher incidence of diabetes when fed A1 beta-casein than when fed A2 beta-casein. Given the statistical significance this was unlikely to be a chance event. The St Bartholomew's mice fed Pregestimil, which contained BCM7, had a higher incidence of diabetes than those fed the soy-based Prosobee. And we also have a level of confirmation from other results from the trial that whole casein (containing a mix of A1 and A2 beta-casein) is diabetogenic.

These results were actually all available within the paper itself, but without explicit information about the contamination of Pregestimil with BCM7, they get lost and overwhelmed in the fog of all the invalid BCM7-confounded treatments.

Actually, I tend to the view that the whole trial was poorly thought out from the start. I think it was Professor Boyd Swinburn (a key figure in Chapter 11) who first pointed out to me that the trial design was much better suited to identifying foods that helped to protect against diabetes, than identifying foods that caused it. Whoever it was that suggested this, I think they were right. The lab animals used were already highly likely to get diabetes. Someone else said to me that they thought the whole FAD trial results should have been thrown away. I think that person was also correct. But what a tragedy. So much time, money and effort and then such a shambles. It is not an easy game!

I admit to being more than a little irritated by the way the confounding in the FAD trial was not openly acknowledged. The presence of Pregestimil in the diets became publicly known back in 2002. It got some limited media coverage, because Pregestimil was supposedly hydrolysed (i.e. proteins broken down into individual amino acids) which would have meant there was no BCM7. Having free BCM7 in a supposedly hydrolysed and hence hypoallergenic infant formula was potentially very serious. Mead Johnson issued a press release saying they had no knowledge of the issue, and would be seeking information from Fonterra. And then it all went quiet. Linking the Pregestimil and BCM7 confounding within the FAD trial was too complex a task for the ordinary news media.

In the pages that follow, as the issues surrounding this trial unfold, I rely heavily on email correspondence, including a lot of direct quotations. I do this to avoid any accusation of 'massaging' the information or quoting it selectively. Instead, I let the people who were involved speak for themselves, exactly as they wrote it in their correspondence with me.

When I became aware of the Pregestimil issues in early 2004 I decided to see what I could do. Sorting out the wheat from the chaff in relation to A1 and A2 beta-casein is difficult enough even when key information is not withheld. And the issue took on greater significance because scientists associated with what seemed to be an anti-A2 campaign kept emphasising how this was an important trial that had failed to confirm the earlier mice trials, and this in turn placed a question mark on whether the epidemiology was sound.

My first foray was in a guest editorial that I had been asked to write on A2 milk for the electronic journal *BioScience News*.[9] I gently pointed out that the main research being used as a counter-argument was the FAD trial, but that 'it is now known that this trial was confounded in several ways, including the presence of beta-casomorphin7 in a filler added to both the A1 and A2 diets.'

Then in *Food New Zealand* the following month I wrote, 'This trial failed to find clear evidence in favour of A2. However, it is now known (although no erratum has been published) that this trial was flawed by a diet filler containing beta-casomorphin7 that was present in both the A1 and A2 diets.'[10]

The Fonterra scientists may have missed the *BioScience News* editorial, although their electronic search-engines should pick up anything with the word 'Fonterra' in it. But they would certainly have seen my comments in *Food New Zealand*, as this is a journal they definitely read. Yet there was no response.

I let things lie for a while in relation to the FAD trial, although I was writing articles for several farming magazines and rural newspapers talking about the need for farmers to give thought to whether they should start breeding A2 cows, and in several of them I referred to the confounding. But then early in 2005 I decided to email Fraser Scott, the corresponding author. The key question I asked him was when did he become aware of the confounding? My assumption was that it must have been after publication, because I could not believe (although I did not state this) that he would knowingly have withheld such information. I received no reply. My email was accepted by the electronic server that houses Fraser Scott's email address, but nothing came back. I have checked many times to make sure that I sent it to the correct address (I have a copy of the email) and I am sure that I did. I cannot of course prove that Fraser Scott read my email, but I am confident that it did get to his electronic mailbox. I emailed again in early 2007, checking once again very carefully that I had his current email address from the Ottawa Health Research Institute (OHRI). The email was accepted by the OHRI server, but again there was no response.

My next step was to write to Bob Elliott, whom I had never met (and still have not met). I explained to him how I had been interested in A2 milk for about 18 months and had written a few articles. Also, that I was now taking things a stage further and writing a book on A2 and associated issues.

I asked Elliott several questions about his work, to which he responded within the hour. But he left the most important question unanswered. This question was: 'I am wondering whether you can shed some light on when the authors other than Jeremy became aware of this confounding.' So I emailed Elliott again, still on the same day (3 Feb 2005):

> What is still not clear to me is whether or not the authors of the FAD trial were aware of the problem with Pregestimil prior to publication. I appreciate that some of the authors may have been suspicious of the results obtained using the Pregestimil base diet, but did Jeremy/NZDRI specifically inform them prior to publication that NZDRI analyses showed there was a high yield of BCM7 from Pregestimil? I have just done a quick internet search and it seems that the Jeremy Hill memo [of 8 October 2000] first got into the media in Nov 2002 which was after publication [of the FAD paper] in *Diabetologia*. It was in Nov 2002 that Mead Johnson released a media statement saying that they were seeking information from Fonterra.

The next morning Elliott responded, 'I can state with certainty that none of the authors were aware of the BCM7 level in the Pregestimil – though both Hubert Kolb and I were concerned about the high diabetes incidence. Furthermore, when I asked Jeremy whether it was possible that the Pregestimil contained BCM7, he said NO.'

My impression from what Bob Elliott wrote was that he had not even been aware of the Jeremy Hill memo of 8 October 2000. This surprised me, but scientists can become so immersed in their own world that these things happen. Since then Elliott has been at the forefront of other work, including transplanting insulin cells from pigs into humans, so he had had plenty of other things to think about. So I emailed him a scanned version of the Hill memo. Within half an hour another email arrived back. Elliott wrote:

> I am still upset by this news. Why did Jeremy do that?? If the Pregestimil used contained BCM7 when the manufacturers state that no peptide [more than] 4 amino acids in length is present in their product, something odd has happened.

> It of course invalidates the Pregestimil arm of the FAD study. This means the two major conclusions of the FAD study are invalid.

So at least on the surface things seemed fairly clear. Of the nine contributing authors only Jeremy Hill apparently knew about the confounding. But there were several more twists in the story yet to come, and things were not as simple as what they seemed. Other authors did indeed know.

Bob Elliott and I agreed that it would be helpful if we could obtain the confidential NZDRI report that Jeremy Hill referred to in his memo. I knew it was highly unlikely that Hill would release it to me, but about three months later I decided to write to him. It took me this long for the simple reason that investigating A2 milk issues is only one of the many things I have to do in life. In the meantime, as well as teaching students at Lincoln University about farm management and agribusiness, I had been working on projects in Papua New Guinea and in Vietnam, plus training for multi-sport (mainly cycling at the time), plus trying with limited success to make some family time. Hill's personal assistant emailed back that he was overseas, but would reply on his return. When no reply came I followed up again and this time, in June 2005, Hill replied: 'Unfortunately the report that you refer to contains information that is confidential to some of Fonterra's customers and as such it will not be possible for me to share this information.'

It was the sort of response I expected. Indeed it is exactly this type of situation, where commercial considerations prevent disclosure of information, that sometimes holds back the advancement of science. But it does seem to fly in the face of claims by Fonterra that 'All the research on this issue [A2 milk] that Fonterra has completed has been published in respected medical or scientific journals, after other scientists who are experts in the field have reviewed it. Fonterra completely rejects any claims by A2 Corporation that it has been secretive.'[11]

I knew that Mead Johnson was not a sponsor of this work (and therefore could not have embargoed the results) but apparently the commercial sensitivities relating to one of Fonterra's business customers meant that the results were to remain hidden.

However, I decided to have another go. I emailed back:

> Thank you for your response. I had hoped that as Mead Johnson were apparently not the sponsors of that work that it would have

> been possible to release the findings. My assumption is that as Pregestimil is supposedly fully hydrolysed protein (or at least that was my understanding) then the presence of BCM7 must have been due to manufacturing quality control problems at that time.

Although I did not state it in my email, I had been made aware by another source that Mead Johnson had recently changed the factory and country of manufacture of the Pregestimil product. This seemed to provide a possible explanation of why things might have gone wrong.

I also asked Hill some other questions relating to his earlier work with A1 and A2 milk, and suggested that some of his criticisms of Corran McLachlan might not be valid.

He then responded that perhaps we should have a meeting, and in early August 2005 we finally got together at Fonterra Innovation in Palmerston North. It was a slightly tense meeting. Hill brought along a Fonterra colleague, Alan Main. I expressed my disappointment that NZDRI/Fonterra Innovation had not admitted to the confounding in the FAD trial. Hill's response was basically along the lines that it didn't really make any difference to the findings. I could only shake my head in amazement. The key facts were very simple: the FAD paper stated that if there was a difference between A1 and A2 beta-casein then it was expected to be because the A1 beta-casein released BCM7 on digestion but the A2 beta-casein did not. It was now known that BCM7 had been included, presumably by accident, in the Pregestimil-based half of the A2 diets, and readers of the scientific paper would inevitably be misled if this information were not reported to them.

We talked for about an hour on various related topics, and in the process I came to understand a little more about Jeremy Hill's perspectives in relation to A1 beta-casein. But basically, there was no meeting of the minds.[12]

My next step was to write to *Diabetologia* reporting the confounding and asking that the paper be retracted from the journal on the grounds of non-disclosure of key information. I asked Bob Elliott if he would co-author this letter, and after some discussion he agreed. Once again the months slipped by with both of us travelling internationally – first me to Brazil and then Bob to Poland – so it was not until late October 2005 that we wrote the letter. We asked for two things: that our letter, which explained in considerable detail the non-disclosure and the background to it, be published in *Diabetologia*; and that the publishers of the journal dissociate themselves from the Beales *et al* paper on the grounds that it had been submitted with key information knowingly omitted.

At this stage events took a very surprising turn. First of all there was an email back from Bob Elliott, who had been contacted by Hubert Kolb. Hubert had been asked by *Diabetologia* for a response to our letter. Bob wrote:

> Although I do not remember anything being discussed about the possibility of the Pregestimil being contaminated with BCM7, Hubert maintains he has an e-mail from me dated about 6 weeks prior to publication that states that I knew BCM7 was in the Pregestimil. If this is the case (and he is an honest man) then I would have to withdraw my comments and co-authorship of your letter. I certainly don't remember this – but that means nothing. I am awaiting a copy of my e-mail to him.

My response was that I too would be interested to see this email. I ventured the opinion that it would probably say that he (Bob) suspected BCM7 in the diets. I reminded Bob that he had been telling me for some months now that he had suspicions about diet contamination. I further ventured the opinion that there was a big difference between his being suspicious based on the trial results, and actual evidence that the diets were confounded. Bob said he hoped I was right, but would have to see what he had actually written some four years earlier.

Then, a few days later came the bombshell in an email from Hubert Kolb to Bob Elliott, which Elliott forwarded to me:

> Please let me repeat the two essential points
> 1. The presence of BCM7 was known to you, me and others before the paper on the FAD trial was published. Your wording in your email at the time the paper was accepted for publication was: 'I hear from Jeremy that the Pregestimil used in the study had peptides >4mers – including BCM7. Apparently all of the current batches have this, unlike earlier (USA derived) batches.'
> 2. The fact that Jeremy had found oligomeric peptides in Pregestimil was discussed at a meeting of the co-authors, including yourself, in London (UK) on September 6-7, 1999. At that time we agreed that

> peptides in Pregestimil may account for the unexpected high background diabetes rate. This left the possibility that a modest effect of A1 vs A2 may have been obscured.

Bob Elliott added, 'The quote is direct from an e-mail I sent to him, so I must withdraw my participation in your letter, as my statement is not correct, and I must accept that my memory is at fault.'

So now we have a completely different situation. Hubert Kolb is saying that he and other authors knew of the confounding prior to publication. Amazing! And if that was the case, how could Bob Elliott have forgotten?

My instincts tell me that Elliott had genuinely forgotten and I think I understand why. He would have been frustrated with many aspects of this trial, including the design of the diets. He also had concerns about diet contamination, and had told me that a staff member from within NZDRI had alerted him that there were 'irregularities in the way the diets were prepared'.

Bob Elliott said that 'we independently examined the diets we were given, and found A1 beta-casein – or at least a protein which migrated on gel electrophoresis in the same spot as A1 in the diet which was supposed to contain A2 only. As this evidence would not stand up in court I have not pursued it further.'[13] He was also unhappy with the way the London group had supposedly worked with the diets. He had told me that 'the London data may have been confounded by that group heating the powders after forming them into cakes, to get rid of water. Glycation end-products caused by heating protein with carbohydrate will cause high diabetes incidence in the NOD mouse.'

In among all of this angst perhaps he had forgotten that he had been made aware of the presence of BCM7. He must have already been heavily disillusioned with many aspects of the trial and also very disappointed at the apparent outcomes. Not only had his own mice died of an infection, but the results from the other labs appeared to support his previous results only partly.

I must admit that I would love to know exactly what Jeremy Hill told his co-authors. How much of the information in the confidential NZDRI report did he share with them? It seems clear that Bob accepted that he must have known something, given the words in his email, but did he know the extent of the evidence?

I have subsequently asked Bob Elliott if Hubert Kolb has supplied him with a copy of the whole email that he (Elliott) wrote. Bob tells me that he has not been supplied by Kolb with a copy of the entire email. Not to ask for it, indeed not to demand to see what he wrote in the context of the total email, seems a little naïve.

One of the problems with having many co-authors can be that what gets written ends up being a compromise. I have little doubt that if Bob Elliott had written the paper it would have looked quite different. In the FAD trial there were nine co-authors and they clearly belonged to different schools of thought in relation to causation of diabetes. For example, Fraser Scott has long been an advocate of cereals as being a causative agent, so perhaps it is not surprising that the paper tended to focus on the differences between the milk diets and the cereal diet, rather than on the difference between the A1 and A2 diets.

Soon after, I received a response back from Professor Edwin Gale, the Editor of *Diabetologia*:

> Thank you for submitting this letter to *Diabetologia*. As you may imagine, it has caused a considerable amount of discussion and concern at this end. Clearly, those best placed to comment on the charges made in your letter are your [sic] co-authors, other than Dr Hill himself. Two of these have now produced lengthy and detailed responses to your allegations, and both profoundly disagree with your conclusions. Because of the potential legal implications of your allegation of scientific misconduct [sic], both our respondents have opted to reserve their statements.
>
> From my own point of view, having read the material submitted to me, and speaking as someone who holds no truck with scientific misconduct, I believe that publication of your letter in *Diabetologia* is not the correct way to take this forward. The normal procedure would be for you to raise your concerns with your [sic] co-authors, and urge retraction of the paper. If this persuasion fails, Professor Elliott still has the option to dissociate himself from the study. I would of course be willing to publish notice of either retraction or dissociation in this journal, but would not consider it appropriate to publish detailed allegations which are contested and currently unsubstantiated.
>
> Should you wish to pursue the charge of scientific misconduct [sic] further, my understanding is that you should produce documentary evidence of this to the institutions sponsoring the studies, or failing this seek legal redress.

Well, there are several issues to take up there. First, Professor Gale made two errors of interpretation: *nowhere* did our letter use the words 'scientific misconduct', and of course, I was *not* one of the co-authors of the paper! How could these misunderstandings arise if he had carefully read what we had written and there had been a 'considerable' amount of discussion about it?

Second – and I would like to be very clear about this – I would never have the temerity to make any suggestion as to whether the apparent knowing non-disclosure involved scientific misconduct, poor judgement or something else. Any claims and judgements on such issues are for others to make. What I am interested in is facts and the progress of science, not judgements about people. All I claim is that important and relevant information was not disclosed; this led (and continues to lead) to scientifically incorrect interpretations in relation to the balance of evidence; *and this situation needs to be remedied.*

Thirdly – and all the more since I was not a co-author – I knew that dealing with the authors was not going to get me very far. I had already had discussions with Jeremy Hill, and two of the other authors (Scott and Kolb) had not responded to my emails. Bob Elliott had been the only one of four authors who was receptive.

The fourth point is that going to the institution sponsoring the study (formerly the NZ Dairy Board, now part of Fonterra) was also not going to get me very far, although I will talk in Chapter 11 about ongoing correspondence with Fonterra in regard to A2 milk. In fact I subsequently made it very clear in emails to Fonterrra CEO Andrew Ferrier that I was very critical of the non-disclosure, but he chose not to respond on that issue. (Because of my position at Lincoln University I am known to most of the senior executives at Fonterra, and I deal with them periodically on a range of issues. But it has been exceptionally hard to get them to engage on issues surrounding A1 beta-casein and A2 milk. In May 2007 I asked Andrew Ferrier when we were going to have a discussion on A2 milk, which I considered to be very important. His response was that even if it were a very important issue he could afford to spend only a very small amount of time on it. I don't think he understands how important it is.)

Accordingly, I wrote back to Professor Gale on 28 November 2005, but this time just in my own name, clarifying various points. The key point in my letter was a request to investigate whether there had been 'non-disclosure of relevant information in relation to confounding, and [had] this led to inappropriate analysis and reporting that [had] the potential to influence scientific thinking.'

Bob Elliott and I had, of course, provided Professor Gale with the key documentary evidence, being Jeremy Hill's confidential memo of 8 October 2000 (Appendix 2). I also provided Gale with copies of all the other relevant correspondence. So it seemed that the investigation was not very complex. But of course it would be controversial, so I suspected that *Diabetologia* would not be keen to get involved.

It took some prodding, but eventually Professor Gale replied:

> Thank you for your reminder of 1st February about this matter, and apologies that I did not acknowledge your email of November 28th. I must confess that I am perplexed as to what you would wish me to do. You were not an author on the original paper, as you point out, and Bob Elliott has agreed that he did have the relevant information before the paper went in.
>
> I am not quite clear as to the way in which the journal is responsible for the accuracy of a statement with which all the authors of a paper appear to agree?
>
> You have asked if *Diabetologia* would be prepared to hold an enquiry into this allegation. The answer to this is a clear 'no'. We do not have the time or the resources to undertake this, and I am still quite unclear as to what you hope to achieve by it. If you believe there is evidence of fraud, this should be presented to the heads of the institutions concerned; I am not aware of any situation in which an academic journal has been asked to take on the task. I am sorry to disappoint you in this way, but have to tell you that I now consider the matter closed.

Well, I think I know when I am getting the brush-off! But I was not totally surprised. Most scientists are aware of examples where journals have taken action in relation to irregularities subsequently discovered in published papers. There again, many people try to avoid controversy, and it can be difficult to get journals to take any action.

I wrote back just one last time to Edwin Gale (who is himself a distinguished professor and researcher in Type 1 diabetes from Bristol University in England). But my email was only very brief, given that Gale had said he considered the matter closed. I suggested he might like to read the editorial in the 24–31 December 2005 issue of *New Scientist* magazine.

So what did this editorial say? It had been penned as a result of a much-publicised cloning scandal involving Woo Suk Hwang of Seoul National University, and was headed 'Breach of Trust'. It stated, among other things, that:

> Science runs on trust. Governments give researchers money on the understanding they will use it fairly and honestly report their results. Peer reviewers assume that what they are judging is a fair account of what happened; they are not yet charged with policing dubious data. Without trust the whole scientific world will collapse.

The editorial also referred to a study by Brian Martinson and colleagues published in *Nature* (Vol 435, p. 727) in 2005. According to the editorial:

> A survey of 3000 researchers funded by the US National Institutes of Health found that 10 per cent or more admitted to withholding details of methodology or results, inappropriately assigning authorship credit, and dropping data points based on gut feeling that they were inaccurate.
>
> So what is to be done? At the very least research ethics need a higher priority both in the education of young scientists and within research institutions. Also, Martinson found that 1 in 8 of his respondents admitted to overlooking other researchers' flawed data or questionable interpretation of data. It is time for scientists to become more active in challenging such instances – as a group of young Korean researchers has done in the Hwang case.

So why didn't the FAD co-authors disclose the information about the confounding? According to Edwin Gale the two co-authors that he contacted produced 'lengthy and detailed responses' but they reserved those statements on account of legal implications. Also, although I have personally written both to Fraser Scott (in January 2005 and again in March 2007) and Hubert Kolb (in November 2005) neither has acknowledged my correspondence. So I can only rely on second-hand accounts from Bob Elliott as to his discussions with Hubert Kolb.

According to Bob Elliott:

> [Hubert Kolb] categorically denied non-disclosure. He referred to a statement on page 1245 of the publication which says 'For example di-(Tyr-Gly) and tripeptides (Tyr Gly Gly) corresponding to the N-terminal fragments of lactalbumin and beta-casein have been shown to have biological activity as do truncated forms of Betacasomorphin.' He states that this was sufficient for an informed reader to draw the conclusion that small peptides were present in the Pregestimil diet. I certainly remember this being discussed at the final meeting of the authors in London – i.e. that peptides up to 4 amino acids in length could be present in Pregestimil. His concerns about the higher than expected rate of diabetes in the Pregestimil group were that a small or modest difference between the two added caseins might have been obscured. These concerns do not appear in the paper. He says that the presence or otherwise of BCM7 doesn't alter the results obtained, and the higher than expected diabetes rate in the Pregestimil group should have alerted readers that there was a diabetogen in that diet. I said that the paper has been used to say that there was no diabetogenic effect of A1 beta-casein – his [Kolb's] reply was that that was a misinterpretation of the data.

I find this all preposterous. It is true that there is a statement in the paper that di- and tri-peptides have biological activity, as do truncated forms of beta-casomorphin, but there is nothing there to say that these were known to be present in the Pregestimil. There is also absolutely nothing in the paper to suggest that BCM7, which is a string of seven amino acids (and hence very different to a di- or tri-peptide, or truncated form of beta casomorphin), was present!

I believe that Bob Elliott summed it up very well in one of his early emails: '*... the two major conclusions of the FAD study are invalid.*'

Earlier in this book I talked about scientists who use statistics for support rather than illumination. It is a human failing, and scientists are very human. We all have a tendency, which as scientists we must fight against, to accept information that fits with our existing viewpoints and to ignore information that challenges an existing perspective. More than 40 years ago Thomas Kuhn wrote a famous book called *The Structure of Scientific Revolutions*. In this he described how new theories that repudiate old theories typically only become mainstream when all the old scientists die off and are replaced by new scientists, without historical baggage, who can look at matters afresh.

In the case of the FAD trial there is no doubt that a number of the authors would have been more comfortable with conclusions that showed casein to be less diabetogenic than cereals, and there is no doubt that finding A1 beta-casein to be diabetogenic would not have been the news that the NZ Dairy Board, by then already part of Fonterra, was hoping for. Did the scientists allow their judgement to be clouded by what they wanted to find out? My guess is that we will never know. But the conduct of the FAD trial has not been good for the advancement of scientific knowledge.

In August 2006 I asked Springer, who are the publishers of *Diabetologia* (and a great many other scientific journals), if they would intervene. The initial response from Gabriele Schroder, the Executive Editor Clinical Medicine at Springer was: 'I have studied the material and have come to the conclusion that Springer as the publisher of the journal *Diabetologia* are not in a position to take any steps to resolve this issue. Edwin Gale, in his capacity as editor-in-chief responsible for the scientific content of the journal, would be the only one to address from your side.'

I responded to Gabriele Schroder that the issues were ethical rather than scientific, and that the final responsibility on ethical issues surely had to lie with the publisher.

I have also suggested to her that Springer, on reflection, might wish to reconsider its position on this matter, and if it were not willing to work with Edwin Gale to resolve this matter in an 'appropriate, professional and ethical manner', that I would like confirmation that their unwillingness to intervene is supported at the highest levels within Springer. This correspondence was also back-copied to Edwin Gale. Schroder's response was to confirm her previous stance (i.e. that it was a scientific matter and out of her hands) and that she had advised the relevant Vice President within Springer of her decision.

I also kept Bob Elliott informed of my actions. Bob showed me a draft of an email to Springer in which he stated as a co-author that he believed there should have been disclosure, and confirmed subsequently that the email had been sent. I note that Springer back-copied to Bob their email response to me, and since I had not given this to them, it is a fairly safe bet that they did indeed receive Bob's email.

So now it is time to move on from the rats and mice. The overall rodent story remains murky. Overall though, it is clear that casein is diabetogenic in these specially-bred diabetes-prone mice and rats. It is also clear that these rodents are susceptible to getting diabetes from a cereal diet. Neither of these points is controversial. The evidence would also seem to be that there is a fundamental difference between A1 and A2 beta-casein in terms of diabetic susceptibility. Bob Elliott's trials demonstrated that very clearly with the NOD mice, and it also seems to be the case with the BB rats in the FAD trial. Fraser Scott and Hubert Kolb have stated that they have further work that is yet unpublished in which they failed to get a difference between A1 and A2 beta-caseins fed to NOD mice. They first made this claim in early 2003 in the *New Zealand Medical Journal*,[14] but more than four years later I can find no evidence in the scientific databases that the paper has been published. And Fraser Scott did not reply to a March 2007 email in which I asked about the publication status. Making claims like this and then not backing them up with publication does not seem to me to be the way science should be conducted. What stopped the publication?

There is one other issue worth considering before finally moving on from the rodents. As I touched on at the start of this chapter, there are actually quite big differences between the different colonies of diabetes-prone rodents. Paolo Pozzilli and colleagues wrote a paper describing some of these differences in different colonies of NOD mice.[15] The NOD mice used at St Bartholomew's certainly had a different underlying susceptibility to getting diabetes than the ones used in New Zealand, and the FAD-trial paper did briefly discuss the possibility that the different colonies might react differently to A1 and A2 beta-casein.

In the greater scheme of things I am not sure that it is crucially important whether A1 beta-casein is diabetogenic in certain groups of rodents. There is so much other evidence relating to humans that perhaps it doesn't really matter what happens with rodents. But it has been impossible for me to ignore the FAD-trial paper when some of its authors (and others such as Professor Truswell) keep bringing it up in various fora as an argument against the A2 hypothesis. When those who are sceptical about A2 milk keep bringing up this so-called evidence, and even claiming as Truswell did in the *European Journal of Clinical Nutrition*[16] that this was an 'important paper ... conducted by a distinguished panel of authors', and that 'any reader of the literature must surely take the findings of experienced researchers in Ottawa, London (England) and Auckland as the latest (perhaps the final) word on this subject', then I have no option but to expose the flaws.

Perhaps the greatest value of the rodent trials is the insights they give into how the scientific game is sometimes played.

NOTES

1 See Elliott and Martin (1984) in Diabetes section of Bibliography.

2 See Elliott *et al* (1997) in Diabetes section of Bibliography.

3 PCT/NZ95/00114, jointly held by the NZ Dairy Board and the National Child Health Research Foundation (NCHRF). The NCHRF subsequently sold its share of this patent to A2 Corporation.

4 See Beales *et al* (2002) in Diabetes section of Bibliography.

5 See Scott and Kolb (2003) in Diabetes section of Bibliography.

6 See Crawford *et al* (2003) and Hill, Boland *et al* (2003) in Heart Disease section of Bibliography.

7 See Truswell (2005) in Industry, Marketing and Overview section of Bibliography.

8 See Truswell (2006) in Industry, Marketing and Overview section of Bibliography.

9 This electronic journal is now defunct. However, the editorial that I wrote remains available on the Lincoln University website. See Woodford (2004b) in Industry, Marketing and Overview section of Bibliography.

10 See Woodford (2004c) in Industry, Marketing and Overview section of Bibliography.

11 This quotation comes from a 12-page document printed on Fonterra letterhead titled 'Briefing paper on the A1 A2 Milk Issue September 2003' that was supplied to interested media both in New Zealand and overseas. There may be more than one version of this document, as my copy contains imbedded file information that indicates that it was modified on 15 June 2004 by Chris Mallett who was Fonterra's Research and Development Director. My copy came to me via American media sources.

12 Much later in early 2007 I wrote to Jeremy Hill seeking confirmation of his position on this matter: 'My understanding of your position was that the non disclosure in the paper made no difference to the overall results. Can you confirm that is a fair summation of your position?' His response was: 'It is some time since I reviewed that work but yes you are correct. I am in Europe at this time so do not have the paper in front of me. The key point was that all milk component containing diets were protective when compared with the non milk containing NPT 2000 diet.' By 'NPT 2000 diet' he was referring to the cereal-based diet that was known prior to the trial to cause a high level of diabetes in these specially-bred rodents.

13 The gel electrophoresis test is not particularly accurate and can show low-level contamination even when there is no contamination. See Huynh *et al* (2006) in Milk and Casomorphins section of Bibliography.

14 See Scott and Kolb (2003) in Diabetes section of Bibliography.

15 See Pozzilli *et al* (1993) in Diabetes section of Bibliography.

16 See Truswell references in Industry, Marketing and Overview section of Bibliography.

CHAPTER SEVEN

THE SCIENCE AND BIG PICTURE OF TYPE 1 DIABETES

If A1 beta-casein is an important risk factor for Type 1 diabetes then there must be biochemical mechanisms (either known or unknown) by which this occurs. It is time to explore what these might be.

I have earlier mentioned Paolo Pozzilli, an Italian scientist who in 1999 reviewed the evidence for milk as a risk factor for Type 1 diabetes. (Pozzilli was also one of the co-authors of the Food and Diabetes trial paper discussed in Chapter 6, but I did not specifically mention him there as his role in that paper was not clear.) His 1999 review included looking at the evidence in relation to individual milk proteins. He concluded that beta-casein was the most promising candidate. He reported results from his own laboratory that 51% of Type 1 diabetes sufferers showed T lymphocytes that were sensitive to beta-casein, versus 2.7% for non-diabetes controls. He also found that 37% of recent-onset Type 1 diabetes sufferers showed antibodies to beta-casein whereas only 5.6% of controls had these antibodies.[1]

Later that same year some German scientists from Frankfurt, led by S. Padberg, published results of tests on both diabetics and non-diabetics for antibodies, not just to beta-casein, but specifically to A1 and A2 beta-casein.[2] They found that the diabetics had high levels of antibodies to the A1 beta-casein, whereas the non-diabetics had higher levels of antibodies to A2 beta-casein. The results were significant at $p < 0.001$, meaning there was greater than 99.9% probability that this result was not just a fluke. They concluded that 'this may confirm the hypothesis of a defective immuno-tolerance to cow's milk in IDDM [Type 1 diabetes].'

In plain language, they were suggesting that diabetics have a defect that causes their bodies to attack something in the A1 beta-casein, after which the body gets muddled and attacks some of its own cells that contain a similar molecule – in this case the cells that produce insulin.

The question of why the body might get confused is an important part of the jigsaw puzzle. To get an answer we need to go back to a patent application that Paolo Pozzilli commenced way back in 1996, and which was finally accepted in 2004 as US Patent 6,750,203. It related to using genetic engineering and/or laboratory removal of beta-casein to produce milk free of non-human beta-casein, in order to provide an 'early infant diet for the prevention of insulin-dependent diabetes'.

The logic behind the patent was that there is a sequence of amino acids (a peptide) in bovine beta-casein that is very similar to an amino-acid sequence within GLUT2, the glucose-transporting molecule inside insulin-producing cells in the pancreas. In fact a sequence of four amino acids (Pro-Gly-Pro-Ile) at one end is identical. Pozzilli was suggesting that this sequence, and larger fragments of beta-casein containing this sequence, 'are responsible for the induction of an immune response towards the casein which, by cross reactivity, would be directed towards the homologous [similar] sequence of GLUT2, causing damage to the cells that produce insulin.'

This common sequence just happens to be identical to the back end of the BCM7 molecule.

When Pozzilli was making his patent application he would have had no evidence that A1 and A2 milk were digested differently. It was only later that this was discovered. So Pozzilli included both A1 and A2 beta-casein in his patent application.

With hindsight it seems likely that Pozzilli got well on the way to making a great discovery, but never quite got there. There is in fact no need to create a new milk by genetic engineering, or to remove beta-casein from the diet. All that is needed is to use A2 cows, which do not produce the A1 beta-casein that breaks down to yield BCM7, which in some people then sneaks into the bloodstream.

So what Pozzilli, and also Padberg and colleagues, are suggesting is that first the body manufactures antibodies to fight the milk devil BCM7, and then by mistake it also attacks the insulin-producing cells in the pancreas because these cells are producing molecules with the same amino-acid sequence as the back end of BCM7.

Now we have a hypothesis that is *really* starting to hang together! To complete the evidence we now need some studies that focus not on antibodies to A1 and A2 beta-casein, but which very specifically focus on BCM7. We need to know whether there is a difference in BCM7 levels in the urine and blood of diabetics – and I am surprised that this work has not already been done.

One of the issues in the past has been that these tests have been difficult to conduct, and a number of laboratories have experienced problems with them. This may be because BCM7 is hydrophobic (water-repellent) and extremely sticky to surfaces like plastic or glass. In other words, if the urine or blood being tested is moved from one flask to another it is very easy to leave the milk devil behind. However, three groups of scientists working on autism and schizophrenia, and who are central to the story told in Chapter 8, seem to be able to conduct these tests successfully. Also, the tests are already available commercially from companies in Norway and the USA.

Unfortunately, however, there is a further complicating issue. In a diabetic the time at which the BCM7 was sneaking into the bloodstream may have been long before the first signs of the disease appeared. In fact, it may have completely passed, leaving no trace, by the time the disease becomes apparent. Indeed, a long delay between time of exposure to the trigger and disease development is common with auto-immune diseases. Therefore the test would need to focus on BCM7 antibodies rather than just on BCM7 itself.

And that creates yet another issue. I am told that measuring antibodies to molecules as small as BCM7 would not be easy. So once again we see that BCM7 is a metaphorical little devil, in that it resists being studied!

It is also not clear whether the 'friendly fire' or 'own goal' hypothesis, whereby the body attacks itself after getting confused between ingested BCM7 and its own GLUT2 molecule, provides the full story. Turning back to non-human animals for a moment, David Chamberlain from the Hannah Research Institute in Scotland led a team of scientists who looked at what happened when beta-casomorphins (including BCM7) were infused directly into the abomasums (part of the rumen) of cattle. They found that the beta-casomorphins lowered the insulin response from the pancreas and believed that this was a direct opioid effect.[3] So maybe our milk devil is multi-pronged.

There are two remaining questions to ask here. The first is whether cereals are an alternative cause of diabetes – after all, there is no doubt that the non-obese diabetic (NOD) mice and Biobreeding (BB) rats get diabetes from a cereal-based diet. The second question is why does the incidence of diabetes keep increasing?

The cereals issue relates to the gluten they contain. Gluten is the main protein in wheat, and is also present in barley and rye, but not corn. It is the constituent of flour that gives bread its elasticity when it rises. There are actually two gluten proteins, glutenin and gliadin. When gliadin is partially digested it can form quite a few opioid peptides, of which the most important is gliadomorphin (also, confusingly, called gliadorphin and gliadinomorphin).

The important point for the current discussion is that gliadomorphin has a very similar structure to BCM7. Both have seven amino acids; both have a tyrosine followed by a proline; both have two further proline molecules in positions 4 and 6. They also have their differences (the full description of gliadomorphin is Tyr-Pro-Gln-Pro-Gln-Pro-Phe), but they are what scientists sometimes refer to as homologous, which is another way of saying 'similar', and there are a number of diseases where it seems that they may be interlinked. Indeed one of the strategies often recommended for reducing the risk of a whole range of auto-immune diseases amongst susceptible people is the gluten-free casein-free (GFCF) diet. In some diseases it appears to be the BCM7 from casein that is the main culprit, while for others such as coeliac disease it is peptides from gluten that take the lead role. In the case of diabetes, the main evidence implicating gluten appears to be some very limited and indeed confusing data suggesting that timing of exposure to cereals may be relevant,[4] plus the undoubted fact that NOD mice and BB rats are extremely diabetes-prone when placed on a cereal-based diet.

Fraser Scott, who was mentioned in the previous chapter in relation to the FAD trial, is undertaking research aimed at identifying human genotypes that are susceptible to cereal-based diabetes. But although it is reasonable to hypothesise that exposure to cereals is a minor risk factor for diabetes, it seems unlikely that it could be a major factor at the population level. Quite simply, the epidemiological data on diabetes in humans is inconsistent with cereals being the major risk factor. And it is also harder to see how the human body could get confused between gliadomorphin and its own insulin-producing cells than is the case for BCM7. This is because the BCM7 molecule more closely resembles the GLUT2 molecule than does gliadomorphin.

The last remaining question we need to consider here is why the incidence of diabetes is increasing. There is no easy answer to this one, but scientists such as Bob Elliott, and Dr Andrew Clarke from A2 Corporation, think the answer may lie in the glycation of BCM7. In 2006

Bob Elliott published a paper on this in the journal *Medical Hypotheses*. Glycation is the process whereby glucose and other sugars react with protein to form sugar-modified proteins called advanced glycation end (AGE) products. There is a huge emerging medical literature showing these are closely linked to a wide range of degenerative diseases. Glycated BCM7 is just one of these AGE products. Levels of glycated BCM7 can be increased by a number of modern food processes including ultra-high-temperature treatment of milk (very common in Europe), the use of ascorbic acid in canned products that have been heated as part of the preservation process, and a generally greater level of sugar drinks consumed by children. Only time will tell if this is the answer.

Reflections on the big picture

All of the known jigsaw puzzle pieces linking A1 beta-casein and BCM7 to Type 1 diabetes have now been presented. Readers now need to make up their own minds as to whether the overall story is convincing. A brief summary of what we know and don't know may help.

We know for sure that there is a much higher rate of Type 1 diabetes in countries where there is a high intake of A1 beta-casein. We know that statistically this is extremely unlikely to be due to a chance event. We also know that if A1 beta-casein is not indeed causative, no-one has been able to produce statistically significant evidence of the actual cause. What we cannot say is that we have 100% proof: we can only talk in terms of very high probabilities.

Animal trials seem to broadly confirm that A1 beta-casein can lead to diabetes. Bob Elliott found that casein diets were diabetogenic in BB rats back in the early 1980s, without knowing which particular component was the cause. Elliott and colleagues then found a very strong relationship between A1 beta-casein and diabetes in their colony of NOD mice. They also found that administration of naloxone, which counteracts the narcotic properties of opioids, stopped diabetes from developing in mice fed A1 beta-casein. Then the FAD trial showed that diabetes-prone BB rats in Canada had a higher rate of diabetes when fed A1 beta-casein in combination with Prosobee than when fed A2 beta-casein in combination with Prosobee, and that this difference was statistically significant. The rest of the FAD trial was a total mess.

Human blood tests indicate that Type 1 diabetics have more antibodies to A1 beta-casein than do non-diabetics, and these results are statistically significant. We also know that the only difference between

A1 and A2 beta-casein is one amino acid in a string of 209, but that this single difference is what causes BCM7 to be formed during the digestion of A1 beta-casein. We also know that the BCM7 molecule formed from A1 beta-casein has a structure very similar to an amino acid sequence in the insulin-producing cells, and this provides a possible explanation of how antibodies attacking the BCM7 could also get confused and attack the insulin-producing cells. And we know that cattle infused with BCM7 have a reduced insulin response.

There are two things we cannot say with confidence. We cannot say whether diabetics have greater levels of BCM7 circulating in their blood than non-diabetics, or (much more importantly) whether they had higher levels of BCM7 circulating at the time the disease was triggered. The reason we cannot say this is that the trials have not been done. Given the time between the triggering of the disease and its appearance, these trials would be very difficult to do. Also, we cannot say with confidence that we know why the incidence of diabetes keeps increasing. All we have is a plausible theory as to why it might be so.

It is also important that people don't get misled into thinking in terms of simple answers, for example that diabetes is caused by one simple factor. Biology seldom works that way. Complex diseases are multi-factorial and hence there are multiple risk factors. So it is highly unlikely that A1 beta-casein is going to provide the total answer. But it is very interesting that diabetes is exceptionally low in the countries that have minimal intake of A1 beta-casein, and moderately low in the countries that have low intake of A1 beta-casein. And it all seems to make sense in terms of the science that we do know, including biochemistry, pharmacology and auto-immune responses. Does this say to us that if we could get rid of the milk devil then a key trigger would disappear? It certainly looks that way to me.

NOTES

1 See Pozzilli (1999) in Diabetes section of Bibliography.

2 See Padberg *et al* (1999) in Diabetes section of Bibliography

3 See Kim *et al* (2000) in Milk and Casomorphins section of Bibliography.

4 See Norris *et al* (2003) in Diabetes section of Bibliography.

CHAPTER EIGHT

AUTISM AND SCHIZOPHRENIA

It is time to move on to look at some new diseases. The focus of this chapter is on autism and schizophrenia.

Autism is a brain disorder that begins in early childhood and persists throughout adulthood. It affects communication and social interaction. People with severe cases may have very poor speech, exhibit temper tantrums and be unable to manage their own toileting. Asperger's syndrome is a relatively mild but common form of autism and many individuals can still operate at a high level. The incidence of autism is debated by experts, with most but not all seeming to agree that the rate has increased greatly in recent decades and that it may be about one child in every 150.

According to the World Health Organisation (WHO) website, schizophrenia is a severe disorder that typically begins in late adolescence or early adulthood. It is characterised by profound disruptions in thinking, affecting language, perception and sense of self. It often includes psychotic experiences such as hearing voices or delusions. It can impair function through the loss of livelihood or the disruption of studies. According to the WHO, there are 24 million suffers of schizophrenia.

Predominantly, this next part of the story involves a totally new set of scientists working in three different countries. The three groups have been led by Professor Robert Cade and Dr Zhongjie Sun from the University of Florida, Paul Shattock from the Autism Research Unit at University of Sunderland, and Dr Kalle Reichelt from the Pediatrics Research Institute at the University of Oslo, Norway. All three groups have interacted with each other and their work is intertwined. Much of it has been published in the journal of *Nutritional Neuroscience*. Other papers have been published in the journals *Brain Dysfunction*, *Autism* and *Peptides*.

First, a brief digression about Professor Robert Cade, who is a nutritional biochemist, now retired, from the University of Florida. One of his best known pieces of work was to design the sports drink Gatorade back in 1965. The Gators were (and are) the University of Florida's football team, and the story goes that they became legendary for their strong second-half performances after drinking the electrolyte-and-energy-replacement drinks concocted by Robert Cade and his wife Mary. Robert's job was to get the appropriate electrolytes and energy balance into the drink; Mary's was to get it to taste acceptable. The royalties from the subsequent commercialisation of this product have been used to finance some of the work on nutritional links to autism that Professor Cade and colleagues have subsequently undertaken. So consumers of Gatorade products can take comfort in the fact that they have contributed to financing some very important work on autism.

Another brief digression. According to a 1998 article in *New Scientist*, Paul Shattock's interest in autism research was originally stimulated by his own experiences as the father of an autistic child.[1] There are several great stories (and I will recount another one in Chapter 9) where a parent's personal experiences in dealing with a particular disease has led to a life-long dedication to finding scientific answers.

The key concept underpinning the work of Reichelt, Shattock and Cade, together with co-workers such as Zhongjie Sun and Ann-Mari Knivsberg, is that many of the symptoms of neurological conditions, i.e. poor mental health, are related to what we eat and how we metabolise that food. Specifically, the symptoms of autism and schizophrenia show some remarkable similarities to the known symptoms caused by opioids which can be formed from the digestion of certain foods, in particular those containing gluten and casein. The particular genetic makeup of an individual, combined with diverse but possibly unrecognised environmental events to which that individual is exposed, determines whether or not that person is susceptible to these conditions. These scientists have been able to show that many autistic children have high levels of BCM7 and other casomorphins derived from BCM7 in their blood and urine. They have also been able to report remarkable success with diets that are free of casein and gluten, in reducing both the level of BCM7 in the urine and the level of autistic symptoms.

The idea that mental health is affected by what we eat has taken a long time to gain acceptance in some medical circles. It has therefore been a difficult journey for Cade, Shattock, Reichelt, Sun, Knivsberg and colleagues. To some extent they were probably ahead of their time, and their contributions to science will be fully recognised only with hindsight.

Until recently these scientists did not realise that BCM7 was released only from A1 beta-casein and not from A2 beta-casein. This is understandable because, as neuroscientists, they did not read the literature on dairy genetics and the ways in which some cows differ from others. So their advice has been, at least until recently, that autistics should consider a diet free of milk. However, there are now at least three different groups of biochemists (including Fonterra's own scientists) who have found that BCM7 is released because of a biochemical feature of A1 beta-casein that is different to A2 beta-casein. So the argument in favour of A2 milk for autistic children comes from linking these separate strands of research.

To the best of my knowledge there have been no trials specifically investigating A2 milk and autism apart from an abandoned trial by Fonterra (and about which I will say more later in this chapter). Instead, research has been focusing directly on the milk devil, BCM7, and similar peptides derived from gluten. However, many parents of autistic children, particularly in Australia where A2 milk has become widely available, are saying that their children's autistic symptoms diminish when their milk intake is restricted to A2. In Britain it is not possible to get certified A2 milk but some parents have been using Guernsey milk, which is very low in A1 beta-casein.

There is also some epidemiological evidence that provides interesting support. Intriguingly, this evidence comes from a patent application by Fonterra, in which they claimed that deaths from mental-health problems were much higher in countries that had high intakes of A1 beta-casein. Subsequently Fonterra abandoned the patent application. This in itself is intriguing and provides a story that I will outline later in this chapter.

The first person to suggest that autism might be linked to opioids was the scientist J.A. Panksepp in a paper published in 1979 in the journal *Trends in Neuroscience*. Then in 1981 Kalle Reichelt and colleagues proposed that these opioids were coming from the incomplete breakdown of certain foods, in particular those containing gluten and casein. Subsequently, the evidence has slowly accumulated that many autistic people do indeed have large quantities of opioids in their blood and urine. There is also evidence that a high proportion of children with autism suffer from increased permeability of the gut wall, and this is a key to explaining what is going on.

Measuring what opioids do in the human body is complex. The method that Reichelt and Shattock use is called High Performance Liquid Chromatography (HPLC), and has gradually been refined but still needs considerable skill. Shattock says that he has now examined more than 1500 autism sufferers and that there are some very clear but complex patterns evident from the chromatography.

At this point a reminder of what a peptide is may be helpful. It is simply a protein fragment. Whereas a protein is made up of many amino acids linked together, a peptide is a much shorter chain of amino acids. Peptides are the first-stage products of protein digestion. The next stage is for them to be broken down into individual amino acids. In most people it is not possible for significant amounts of peptides to get through the gut wall into the bloodstream. But for other people with so-called 'leaky guts' these peptides can get through the gut wall.

A key point in relation to autism and schizophrenia is that the gliadomorphin from gluten and the BCM7 from milk seem to 'hunt together'. Readers may recall from Chapter 7 that they have a very similar structure. With coeliac disease (which will be discussed in Chapter 9) it is clear that gluten and its derivatives play the lead role. Any role played by BCM7 is subsidiary. However, in the case of heart disease it would seem that the milk devil, BCM7, acts independently of any involvement by gluten. And in the case of Type 1 diabetes, although it seems that the milk devil plays the prime role, it would be foolish to totally discount the potential importance of gluten. In autism and schizophrenia it seems that metaphorically speaking, the gluten and the casein stand shoulder to shoulder in their attack.

One of the more important papers linking gluten and casein to autism and schizophrenia was published by Robert Cade and seven co-authors in *Nutritional Neuroscience* in 2000, and titled 'Autism and Schizophrenia: Intestinal Disorders'. Their starting point was Dohan's hypothesis from way back in 1966: that schizophrenia is linked to gluten consumption from wheat, barley, oats and rye. That hypothesis stemmed from the observation that schizophrenia was very rare and mild in societies where these grains were not used, but very common and severe in countries where they made up a large part of the diet. The hypothesis was later extended to include milk.

Cade and his colleagues then asked the following six questions:

1 Is there an unusually high concentration of peptides in blood and urine of schizophrenic and autistic patients?

2 If [peptides] enter the blood, can they penetrate the blood/brain barrier?
3 What structures do they enter?
4 Could involvement of the brain structures the peptides enter cause the symptoms of autism and schizophrenia?
5 If the peptides are removed or greatly decreased in concentration are the disease symptoms and signs diminished or cured?
6 If a normal animal is given one of the peptides will it produce symptoms similar to those of autism and schizophrenia?

For all six questions there was in fact already published evidence suggesting an affirmative answer, and Cade and his colleagues laid out the sources of this information. But they pointed out that no one team of scientists had previously attempted to join all these questions together. In doing this, they also presented extensive previously unpublished data they had collected from 150 autistic children and 120 schizophrenic adults. They also included data from 76 normal adults and 43 normal children.

The story they found is quite complex (very seldom are there simple answers in medicine) but the answers were also very clear. Normal subjects had three different patterns of peptide excretion, with each individual fitting into one category. The autistic children and schizophrenic adults exhibited the same three patterns, but with much greater levels of peptide excretion. In fact there was no overlap in the ranges, with perfect separation for each pattern type between on the one hand those with autism and schizophrenia, and on the other hand those who were normal controls. So yes, there *was* an unusually high concentration of peptides in the blood and urine of these schizophrenic and autistic patients.

They also found that more than 85% of all autism and schizophrenia sufferers had greatly enhanced IgG antibodies to casein and gluten. IgG antibodies are part of the body's immune system. The greatly enhanced sensitivity of these antibodies to gluten and casein in autism and schizophrenia sufferers strongly suggests that the body is trying to fight something related to these peptides.

Perhaps the most interesting data relate to what happened when autism sufferers were placed on a diet free of any casein and gluten. Of 70 autistic children ingesting a gluten-free casein-free (GFCF) diet, and who were followed for one to eight years, 81% improved significantly within three months on a range of scores such as social isolation, eye contact, mutism, learning skills, hyperactivity, stereotypal activity, panic attacks and self-mutilation. Of the 13 children who did not improve, five continued to excrete high levels of casomorphins and gliadomorphins, suggesting they may not have been following the prescribed diet.

For schizophrenia sufferers the success rate was only 40%. A major problem here was that most of those who did not respond quickly subsequently failed to stick with the diet. And this is one of the key problems with GFCF diets: the response is not immediate and in the first few weeks it may in fact be quite negative owing to opioid withdrawal symptoms. However, for those who do persist and get a positive response, the improvement is ongoing for at least 12 months. It seems that it may take at least that long to get all of the BCM7 off the opiate receptors in the brain. Those who then go off the diet typically regress.

Another important paper published in *Nutritional Neuroscience* the following year (2001) was by the Norwegians Ann-Mari Knivsberg, Kalle Reichelt and M. Nodland. They summarised a series of trials and dietary interventions that they had undertaken with autism sufferers over a period of 12 years. Their data included both groups and individuals. They concluded:

> People with autism are as different from each other as people without development disorders are. Dietary intervention is no cure that can remove all autistic traits in all children with autism. There can be no doubt, though, that the vast majority of the participants described were more harmonious, more social, communicative and capable of using his or her skills in a better way than before the diet was implemented. The reports thus should form a solid basis for further investigations on the effect of dietary intervention in autism.

Ann-Mari Knivsberg and Kalle Reichelt have continued to publish regularly, sometimes with co-authors. In 2002 they published a paper in *Nutritional Neuroscience* titled 'A Randomised, Controlled Study of Dietary Intervention in Autistic Syndromes'.[2] In the abstract they stated that 'A randomly selected diet and control group with 10 children in each group participated. Observations and tests were done before and after a period of one year. The development for the group of children on diet was significantly better than for the controls.'

This trial was 'investigator-blind', meaning that although the parents of the children knew the type of diet their child was on, the investigators who were taking the measurements did not know. Currently this appears to be the only trial of the GFCF diet that has involved a control group and has been investigator-blind.[3]

A major challenge with investigating the GFCF diet is to meet the desired scientific standard of 'double blind'. One suggested approach is to have both the trial group and the control group (both of which would comprise autistic children) on a GFCF diet, and then for each group to be given a supplement that was either free of casein and gluten, or rich in these proteins. A variation on this is to use the 'crossover' approach, where halfway through the trial the GFCF group shifts to the casein-and-gluten supplement and vice-versa. Once again, the only people who would know who is getting which supplement would be scientists who are totally independent from the trial except for holding the diet codes. This protocol has recently been tested for a 12-week period (6 weeks plus 6 weeks) on 15 children, 12 of whom completed the test.[4] But to get meaningful results the trial would need much larger numbers of children and to be conducted for much longer, because of the time taken for the opioid peptides to be eliminated from the brain and for measurable impacts on development to show up. As of April 2007 a group from University of Rochester Medical Centre, New York, was recruiting for a similar preliminary trial with 30 children.[6] Yet another group from the University of Pittsburgh has a similar trial planned using 80 children, but for the longer time of three months per treatment.[5] Even then, the Pittsburgh team describe its work as only phase 1. It says that 'Phase 1 data will be used to obtain funding for double-blind trials (phase 2) and the study of neurobiological mechanisms underlying improvement in symptoms (phase 3).' Hopefully, the three month treatment will be long enough to identify any changes that are occurring, but it is still a short time period given the findings of Cade and his colleagues.

So it is going to be a long time before there are any results from GFCF diets that classically trained scientists who demand controls and double-blinding might regard as proof. And there are still likely to be many challenges along the way with children dropping out of these artificial diets. Most drug companies, which are working with products like pills that are logistically much simpler than a whole diet, base their plans on the assumption that it takes at least 10 years to get a new product to market after the first promising results are obtained. So it could well take as long or longer to get conclusive results from the GFCF diets.

In the absence of proof from double-blind diet trials it is inevitable that there should be a focus on individual case studies and anecdotal reports. In fact there are many thousands of people who follow the GFCF diet. American scientists George Christison and Kristin Ivany have noted that in 2005 there were nine discussion groups on yahoo.com alone devoted primarily to this topic, with a combined membership of over 10,000.[7] Also, they say that the website gfcfdiet.com supports 180 'Autism and GFCF Diet' support groups in the USA alone.

Some scientists tend to be very critical of case histories and observational reports on the grounds that they are anecdotal and hence do not have the controls that rigorous scientific research regards as so important. Undoubtedly, some believers will be influenced by wishful thinking and not all such 'evidence' will be valid. Nevertheless, I have chosen to quote from one of them because they provide information about the fabric of decisions that every parent of an autistic child has to make. There are numerous such reports posted on the web, but I have chosen to quote here from the website of Jorgen Klaveness, a Norwegian lawyer. There is something particularly moving about the way that he writes:

> When my son was 18 months old, he started to slip away from us. He was diagnosed with a 'brain disorder', later he got the 'autistic label'. Those of you who have been through the same process know what he went through.
>
> At a certain stage, we stopped wondering if something was wrong with our child, and started looking for what we could do for him. We stopped being afraid that he might be an idiot, and started marvelling at the way the little chap was, in his own way, struggling along with his enormous problem.
>
> When he was eight years old, we heard about the GFCF diet. We're lucky to live in Norway, close to one of the foremost research centres in the world, and to Dr Karl Ludvig Reichelt ... After a short trial period, we've never looked back without shuddering at the idea of what would have happened if we hadn't met Dr Reichelt ... We've never got 'back' the son we hoped for initially; he'll never be able to make up for all that he lost during his first eight years. But his entire life has been taken up in a new direction. He's able to learn again. He has learnt to speak. He plays with other children. He's become toilet trained. He has developed a strong sense of humour and a genuine attachment to us. He means something for us and we mean something for him. We're connected ...
>
> I want as many as possible of the world's autistic children to have

> the chance that my son got when he was eight. I also want as many of them as possible to get the chance that he didn't get when he was two.

Klaveness also wrote about the problems of getting repeated double-blind crossover experiments of the type that are generally accepted as scientific proof:

> That kind of proof isn't likely to appear in the next few years either. The experiment would be costly and very time consuming, and the treatment is relatively simple, cheap, and available without a prescription. Nobody is going to make money out of it, and therefore too little research is likely to go into it.

Perhaps Klaveness was not quite right when he said the treatment was simple. Many people find that sticking to a diet free of gluten and casein is in fact very difficult. Not only is there ongoing temptation to give in, but there are many foods that must be avoided and many hidden sources of gluten and casein. Klaveness himself reports how his child for a long time continued to have an intake of gluten from supposedly gluten-free foods.

A further comment from Klaveness also seems relevant:

> As parents of autistic children, we don't need scientifically tested hawsers. We'll throw our children any piece of string or straw that offers hope. The GFCF diet is such an option. Our experience tells us that it will work for some. We believe that it will work for many. It is likely to work better the earlier you start.

Despite the lack of double-blind trials of a GFCF diet there is of course considerable scientific evidence relating to beta-casomorphins and autism. The associations that Cade, Sun, Reichelt and Shattock have all found between peptides in the urine and autism are hard to dismiss. However, other scientists using other methods have not as yet been able to replicate their results and so the methods remain controversial.[8]

So far in this chapter I have placed considerable focus on gluten and casein in combination. The human trials and dietary interventions that have been reported have in general not tried to separate one from the other. The justification for this has been the assumption that opioid peptides from both gluten and casein are being absorbed into the bloodstream, and then crossing the blood/brain barrier. However, it is now time to look more carefully at what we know about BCM7 independent of any combined effects with peptides from gluten. This work comes from animal trials.

Zhongjie Sun and Robert Cade undertook some very informative work where they injected BCM7 into rats. In one such trial, published in the journal *Autism* in 1999, they used BCM7 to investigate to which parts of the brain, if any, the BCM7 became attached. To measure the outcomes they had to euthanise the rats and dissect the brains. The answer they obtained was that the BCM7 became attached to areas of the brain that had 'been shown to be altered either functionally or anatomically in patients with schizophrenia, and most have been shown to be functionally abnormal in autism.' They concluded that BCM7 could cross the blood/brain barrier, activate opioid receptors and affect brain regions similar to those affected by schizophrenia and autism.

In another trial, also published in *Autism* in 1999, Sun and Cade injected normal rats with BCM7 to investigate their subsequent behaviour. Cade and his co-authors referred to this work in their *Nutritional Neuroscience* paper of 2000:

> Fifty seven seconds later the rats began running frantically, knashing their teeth and foaming at the mouth. They then became hostile and defensive, attacking their normal cage mate if it came near. Pain sensitivity was greatly decreased, a finding occurring frequently in many patients with autism and schizophrenia. They also paid no attention when a bell was rung over their cage while normal rats invariably looked up for the source of the sound. This is of interest because mothers of children with autism frequently think their child is deaf.

Sun and Cade reported in the journal *Peptides* in 2003 that in normal rats, gliadorphin (GD7), the major opioid in gluten, affected only three regions of the brain, while BCM7 affected 45. Also, they demonstrated that the mechanism by which GD7 gained access to brain cells was by 'diffusion through circumventricular organs', while BCM7 passed the blood/brain barrier by 'carrier facilitation'.

In other words, the GD7 can only get into a few bits of the brain by sneaking through the bushes whereas BCM7 drives straight up the highway and goes wherever it wants to. Also, they noted that BCM7 caused 'bizarre behavior changes' whereas GD7 caused no behavioural change.

Earlier in this book I explained how the milk devil BCM7 is released on digestion of A1 beta-casein but not from A2 beta-casein. It is now time to look at what happens in relation to autism and schizophrenia when people consume A2 rather than A1 milk.

Back in 2001 the New Zealand Dairy Research Institute (NZDRI), at that stage still part of the NZ Dairy Board but about to become part of Fonterra, the world's largest international trader of dairy products, applied for a patent concerning A1 beta-casein, autism and schizophrenia.[9] The patent application was titled 'Milk containing beta-casein with proline at position 67 does not aggravate neurological disorders'. In plain language that means A2 milk does not aggravate mental health disorders. The Abstract then says:

> The invention is based on the discovery that the consumption of milk which contains a beta-casein variant which has histidine or any other amino acid not proline at position 67, may on digestion cause the release of an opioid which may induce or aggravate a neurological/mental disorder such as autism or Asperger's syndrome. The invention is supplying milk or milk products that contain beta-casein with proline at position 67 to susceptible individuals.

In other words the NZDRI was claiming that ordinary milk containing A1 beta-casein caused or aggravated mental disorders such as autism, and that susceptible individuals should consume only A2 milk. The five inventors were listed as Robert Crawford, Michael Boland, Carmen Norris, Jeremy Hill and Robin Fenwick. Readers may remember some of these names from earlier chapters of this book. But what a bombshell!

The evidence they produced in support had four parts to it. One was theoretical, in relation to the opioid characteristics of BCM7. This was well known and not controversial, and in itself was not patentable. The second part was that BCM7 was released from A1 beta-casein (and other variants not having proline at position 67) but not from A2. This also was confirmatory rather than new, as it had previously been reported from both German and Japanese laboratories. Whereas the German and Japanese papers were unequivocal on this matter, the NZDRI patent application was not quite so sure, and said:

> The levels of BCM7 measured in hydrolysis of A2 casein were far less than that measured in the hydrolysis of A1 casein. It is difficult to tell, however, due to the presence of small quantities of A1 casein in the A2 casein, whether the BCM7 was formed from the hydrolysis of the A2 casein or to a small amount of A1 casein contaminant, or both. If BCM7 was formed from the hydrolysis of A2 casein, the rate of reaction was many orders of magnitude less than that observed with the hydrolysis of A1 casein.

My bet is that the small release apparent from A2 casein was indeed due to A1 contamination, and that the German and Japanese scientists got it right. It is frustrating that so many of the A2 diets manufactured by NZDRI seem to have been contaminated.

The third part of the evidence was a trial with autistic and non-autistic (control) children aged 6–18 years. Some autistic children were given A2 milk after overnight fasting and then showed low levels of casomorphins in their urine, while others given A1 milk showed up to a 10-fold increase in casomorphins. For normal children (age-matched controls) there was no such increase. This was consistent with results obtained by Cade, Reichelt and Shattock, but it was also new in that this was the first time that A1 and A2 beta-casein had been compared directly.

The fourth part, which was totally new, was the epidemiology. The NZDRI team was able to find 10 developed countries for which there was both satisfactory information on A1 beta-casein intake and data on death rates attributable to mental disorders. The countries were Australia, Canada, Denmark, Finland, Germany, Iceland, New Zealand, Norway, Sweden, and the USA (data from San Diego). The source of death-rate data was the WHO.

The results were staggering! They found that 63% of the between-country variation in deaths from mental conditions can be explained statistically by differences in the intake of A1 beta-casein. The probability of getting a result like this by chance is 0.006 (less than one in 160). In contrast the relationship between A2 beta-casein intake and deaths from mental disease was negative but not statistically significant. This means it would not be valid to claim that A2 is actually protective, but rather that it has no proven influence either way.

The NZDRI team re-ran the analysis with Iceland excluded, on the grounds that Iceland had a low incidence of mental disease and presumably looked as though it might be anomalous despite also having milk that is low in A1 beta-casein. But this produced an even higher correlation between A1 intake and mental disease. The NZDRI team also separated out males and females but this provided no new insights, with similar outcomes for both sexes.

So how should we interpret these results? We cannot say with absolute certainty that A1 beta-casein causes deaths from mental illness, because we can never get absolute proof from any correlation. But we can say that the probability of getting a result like this through chance is highly unlikely. It is an amazing result.

These results have never been published in the scientific literature. In fact it wasn't too long before the NZDRI, now part of Fonterra, abandoned the patent application. The reasons subsequently reported in the news media were that they had undertaken follow-up trials with autistic children and were no longer able to obtain the BCM7 peaks in the urine. However, the truth would seem to be not quite that simple.

I did my own little bit of exploration in regard to those subsequent trials and managed to track down one of the scientific investigators involved in them. He was happy to explain the situation to me on the telephone. My file notes from that conversation (in August 2004) state that the trial involved 18 autistics and 18 non-autistics who were age-matched. The trial was a double-blind crossover trial in which participants were fed milk (either 'ordinary', i.e. mixed A1 and A2, or straight A2) and urine samples were collected four hours later. The crossover took place four weeks later. Each sample was then split in two, of which one was analysed at Auckland University and the other at NZDRI in Palmerston North. The analyses showed 'lots of noise in the system, with not only high variance but inconsistent results from split samples'. Whoops! Inconsistent results from split samples meant the analysts in Auckland were getting different results from those in Palmerston North for exactly the same sample. Something was wrong with the testing procedures and so the whole trial had to be abandoned. But that is quite different to saying there were no differences between the autistics and non-autistics.

There are a number of reasons why this trial might have gone astray, but an obvious contributing factor is poor technique in at least one laboratory. As explained in Chapter 7, BCM7 is tricky to analyse for. There may also have been other flaws, including A1 and A2 contamination.

Some other A2 diets supplied by NZDRI around that time are known to have been contaminated with A1 beta-casein, including the samples used for digestion trials of the release of BCM7 in human subjects. Another example of this was presented in Chapter 4. Alternatively, the equipment may not have been properly set up and calibrated in at least one of the labs. But we will never know. The trial was buried and Fonterra abandoned the patent.

But what about the epidemiology? Presumably those results still stand? The scientists couldn't just make up the analyses, and the applicants for the patent would have had to sign documents stating that the application was based on truthful knowledge. The answer is indeed yes, those results do stand. So we cannot simply ignore them and pretend they do not exist. They have not been repudiated.

I have gone back to the WHO databases and undertaken some preliminary correlation analyses, which confirm that statistically significant relationships do exist, although for the year that I investigated (2000) the relationships were not as strong as those found by the NZDRI scientists. The relationship also holds with a larger sample of countries, using the Laugesen and Elliott A1 beta-casein consumption data. But just how we should interpret these results is problematic. For a start, the NZDRI calculations (and my own) were quite crude. If a country has a low birth rate compared to other countries, its overall death rate will be higher simply because old people make up a larger part of the population. (This is why people such as Murray Laugesen and Bob Elliott, and also Corran McLachlan, use age-related rates, such as the death rate in a particular age class.) Did this create a bias? Perhaps. This sort of bias usually creates a meaningless picture (a 'fog') rather than a deceptive one (a 'mirage'). Also, people who suffer from diseases such as schizophrenia do not necessarily die directly from it. So how reliable are these statistics? There is no simple answer to this and related questions. All we can say is that even if we cannot understand and readily explain such results we should be cautious of rejecting them as supposedly due to random factors, given their statistical significance. Ignoring results that we do not like and do not understand is quite common, but it is not good science.

So here we have yet another area of research that needs to be followed up.

While pondering on these issues I decided to explore the recorded causes of death of people suffering from schizophrenia. The answers were fascinating. There have been quite a few studies done and they all seem to show broadly similar results. Schizophrenia sufferers not only have significantly increased death rates from suicide (which in previously identified schizophrenics are likely to be recorded as due to schizophrenia), but they also have considerably increased death rates from natural causes, especially cardiovascular disease (more than twice the rate).

What is this saying to us? Can it be explained by the lifestyle these people lead? Or is it linked to a leaky gut? If schizophrenics do indeed typically have a leaky gut leading to BCM7 passing through into their bloodstream (and the evidence from Cade, Sun, Reichelt and Shattock seems to be compelling on that) could this explain, in line with the evidence of Chapters 3 and 4, why they would also have increased deaths from cardiovascular disease? There is certainly lots to think about!

New pieces of the jigsaw puzzle continue to be found, although deciding where they fit into the big picture can be problematic. For example, in 2006 Kalle Reichelt and O. Skjeidal reported in the journal *Autism* that IgA antibodies to casein have been found in girls with Rett syndrome.[10] They stated their analyses on 23 sufferers were statistically 'highly significant' in comparison to 53 normal persons used as controls.

Rett syndrome is a serious neuro-developmental disorder caused by a genetic mutation. Reichelt and Skjeidal suggest that their results indicate increased peptide uptake from the intestines by people with this syndrome. The implications of this are that although the fundamental problem is genetic, one of the outcomes may be increased permeability of the intestines (leaky gut) which in turn leads to increased uptake of peptides from gluten and casein. This then causes or exacerbates some of the neurological symptoms. Other studies have shown that gastrointestinal disorders are indeed very common in people with Rett syndrome.

Another piece recently fitted into the puzzle is a 2006 paper in a Norwegian journal by E. Sponheim and colleagues, including Reichelt.[11] They found in a small group of high-functioning autistics that only three out of 17 had abnormal peptides in the urine (compared to no abnormal peptide levels in healthy unrelated controls). This contrasts with the much higher levels of abnormality that Cade, Reichelt and Shattock found for more seriously affected autistics.

The big picture

It is now time to summarise the big picture in relation to autism and schizophrenia. It is apparent that many autistics and schizophrenics excrete abnormally high levels of BCM7 and other similar peptides in their urine. This declines markedly when these people are placed on a gluten-free and casein-free diet. The investigations by teams led by Cade, Reichelt and Shattock in three different countries confirm this.

We also know that BCM7 is released by the digestion of A1 beta-casein, but is either not released at all, or only in tiny amounts, from A2 beta-casein.

Numerous investigations show that eliminating casein and gluten from the diet leads to a marked improvement in the symptoms of autism. Once again Cade, Reichelt and Shattock stand to the fore, together with Reichelt's colleague Ann-Mari Knivsberg. However, none of these medium- to long-term trials has been undertaken using double-blind protocols. Such trials are exceptionally difficult to conduct, but several are being planned. There is one published trial with significant results where the investigators were blind, and several other trials where they were not.

We also know that when BCM7 is injected into rats it causes them to act in a bizarre fashion, with many symptoms that resemble autism. Also, that the BCM7 enters many areas of the brain that are linked to autism, whereas similar peptides from gluten cannot access most of these areas.

We know that many thousands of parents of autistic children use a GFCF diet and believe it has benefits, but we also know that individual case studies such as this are not necessarily reliable.

We also have unsolicited testimonials supplied to A2 Corporation by parents of autistic children who have been given A2 milk. These parents believe their children are better on A2 milk than ordinary milk.[12] Once again, these are only observational case histories that lack controls. However, these results seem plausible, in that we know there is unlikely to be a release of BCM7 from A2 milk.

There are also other pieces to the puzzle, such as the unpublished epidemiological results obtained by Fonterra's scientists, and the published finding of elevated casein antibody levels in Rett syndrome sufferers. Just where these pieces of evidence fit into the overall picture, or whether they do have a place, is yet to be determined.

In the final analysis, readers will have to make up their own minds whether the overall story is convincing.

A final issue to consider and clarify is whether opioids such as those from beta-casein and gluten are causing the *syndromes* of autism and schizophrenia or whether they are causing or exacerbating the *symptoms* of these syndromes. The syndrome, or underlying condition, may well be genetic in origin, with only some human genotypes being susceptible. However, the symptoms either only appear, or else are greatly exacerbated, when BCM7 is absorbed into the bloodstream through the intestines and then manages to get across into the brain. So although the opioids may not be the fundamental problem, they do irreversible damage in susceptible people. That is why people like Jorgen Klaveness talk of the importance of an early start with dietary intervention.

NOTES

1 *New Scientist* v158.n2139(June 20, 1998); pp42–45.

2 See Knivsberg *et al* (2002) in Autism and Schizophrenia section of Bibliography.

3 A detailed review of existing scientific studies of the GFCF diet is provided in Christison and Ivany (2006). See Autism and Schizophrenia section of Bibliography.

4 See Elder *et al* (2006) in Autism and Schizophrenia section of Bibliography.

5 See U.S. National Institutes of Health clinical trials database, www.clinical trials. gov/ct/show/NCT100090428?order=1. Accessed 25 April 2007.

6 Accessed from the UCLID Centre of the University of Pittsburgh website. www. uclid.org:8080/uclid/re_autism.html. Accessed 25 April 2007.

7 See Christison and Ivany (2006) in Autism and Schizophrenia section of Bibliography.

8 See Dettmer *et al* (2007) in Autism and Schizophrenia section of bibliography. This paper reports an inability to find these urinary peptides using an online HPLC method. However, other scientists are questioning this methodology.

9 The patent application number under the International Patent Application Treaty is WO 02/19831 A1 and is dated 14 March 2002. The application also carries the earlier NZ identifier of PCT/NZ01/00186.

10 See Reichelt and Skjeidal (2006) in Austism and Schizophrenia section of Bibliography.

11 See Sponheim *et al* (2006) in Autism and Schizophrenia section of Bibliography.

12 See A2 Corporation website, www.a2corporation.com

CHAPTER NINE

ALLERGIES, INTOLERANCE AND AUTO-IMMUNITY

Nearly everyone seems to know someone who is either allergic to or intolerant of milk. But what does this actually mean? What is the difference between allergy and intolerance? What is causing these reactions? Is it possible or likely that BCM7 from A1 beta-casein is in some way involved? Is there a link between milk allergies and a range of auto-immune conditions? These are the issues I will explore in this chapter.

The word 'allergy' was coined in 1906 by an Austrian paediatrician, Clemens von Pirquet, who used it to describe responses in his patients to various agents such as dust, pollen and certain foods. But the term did not come into widespread use until the 1950s. What we now know is that allergies are set off by the presence of allergens (also called antigens). Typically these are proteins of various types. Although they are not normally harmful in themselves, the body gets tricked into believing that they are harmful and so it sets out to attack them. It does this by producing antibodies, in particular what are known as IgE antibodies (also called IgE immunoglobulin) which try to attach themselves and thereby smother the apparent external invader. In the process there can be a large release of a substance called histamine. The histamine may in turn cause a range of conditions such as hives or asthma, and in severe cases even anaphylactic shock and death. There is no doubt that in some people milk causes these reactions, but there are also many other foods and toxins that can create these effects. Indeed it seems that there may be very few proteins, perhaps none, that are totally non-allergenic for all people.

Milk intolerance is different. A person who is intolerant of milk, or one of its constituents, will typically experience bloating and/or diarrhoea. Some people may experience constipation before the diarrhoea. Whereas allergies are typically a response to proteins, intolerance may be due to either proteins or other food components. For example, lactose intolerance is caused by an inability to digest lactose (milk sugar) on account of a deficiency of the enzyme lactase. Although this is the most widely accepted form of milk intolerance, we shall see as this chapter progresses that sometimes a supposed lactose intolerance may in fact be due to something else in the milk. No prizes for guessing what this might be!

In practice, the distinction between an allergy and intolerance can get blurred. To a scientist the distinction is quite clear: allergies involve immune responses via antibodies; intolerance does not. But allergies and intolerance sometimes run together. If the body is allergic to a particular protein then the gut may well join the party and empty out with great rapidity as part of the response mechanism.

Whereas an allergy is a response to an externally sourced protein, (e.g. ingested in food, inhaled into the lungs or simply by skin contact), an auto-immune condition occurs when the body attacks and destroys particular types of its own cells. How does the body get fooled into taking this destructive action? After all, there are more than 40 recognised auto-immune diseases, and many more diseases that are suspected of having an auto-immune component. According to the American Autoimmune Related Diseases Association (AARDA) about 20% of Americans suffer from auto-immune conditions.[1]

Why is the body so stupid as to attack itself? At this stage science has no simple answers. But the generally accepted view is that some external agent – be it a disease, a type of food or a toxin – sets the body off down this false trail. In essence, the body gets confused between the external agent and its own cells.

With most or perhaps all auto-immune diseases there is a genetic component. We should therefore choose our parents with care! But if heredity primes the gun, it still takes one or more environmental factors to pull the trigger.

In the early years, A2 Corporation made no claims whatsoever in relation to A2 milk having benefits for people with milk intolerance or allergies. But then, from early 2003, when A2 milk first came on the market in New Zealand and Australia, consumers kept coming back to A2 Corporation with stories about how they could digest A2 milk, whereas they could not digest A1 milk. Many of these endorsements are on the A2 Corporation website. Also, there were several items on Australian current-affairs television programmes, with people praising the benefits of A2 milk in relation to all sorts of medical conditions. One such programme called it 'Wonder Milk'.

Almost certainly these endorsements came as no surprise to Corran McLachlan, who at that time was still the Chief Executive Officer of A2 Corporation. I am told by a friend of his that McLachlan was himself intolerant to ordinary milk but that he could drink A2 milk.

Some of the endorsements that have come back to A2 Corporation are from people who had previously considered themselves to be lactose intolerant. However, there is no obvious reason why lactose intolerance should be less of a problem with A2 milk than ordinary milk. It is possible that the BCM7 in ordinary milk slows down the excretion of waste products from the body, because opioids definitely can have this effect on some people. And it is well known that there is something in casein that causes this slowing-down effect (see Chapter 2). This would provide more time for the undigested lactose to ferment and cause problems. But this is nothing more than a hypothesis that is logical but totally untested in scientific trials. Another possibility is that a number of people considered to be lactose intolerant have in fact been misdiagnosed. Given the nature of the common tests for lactose intolerance this is very plausible.

I will recount just two anecdotes of my own, although I do have others.

Back in November 2004 there was a feature article in the Christchurch newspaper, *The Press* about Crohn's disease and ulcerative colitis. Both of these diseases involve severe inflammation of parts of the intestinal tract. The main thrust of the article was to explore the potential link between these debilitating diseases and a wasting disease in cattle called Johne's disease (pronounced 'Yo-knees'). Johne's disease is caused by a bacterium, *Mycobacterium paratuberculosis*, or MAP for short. A link between MAP and Crohn's, and also ulcerative colitis, has been suspected for about 20 years but has been difficult to pin down.

Alongside this article there was the case history of Claire, a lady who suffered from Crohn's disease. Claire was also President of the Canterbury Crohn's and Colitis Support Group. She described the way it affected both her lifestyle and what she could eat. She explained that among other things she had cut out all dairy products except for the occasional 'cheese toasty'. According to the website of the Crohn's and Colitis Support Society about 35% of Crohn's sufferers and 20% of ulcerative colitis sufferers cannot tolerate milk.

I already knew Claire (although not very well) and I cut out the article, and over the next few weeks I read and re-read it several times. As an agriculturalist I already knew a moderate amount about Johne's disease, and the possible link with Crohn's disease. I also realised that both Crohn's and ulcerative colitis increased the chances of a person having a leaky gut that would facilitate passage of peptides into the bloodstream. For a while I did nothing, as I told myself that it was none of my business. But every so often the article would emerge from the pile of papers strewn around my office and I kept thinking, 'I reckon Claire might have a susceptibility to A1 beta-casein.' It took me more than three months to do anything, but eventually I sent her an email:

> I have been meaning to contact you since seeing an article in the paper about you.
>
> You may like to see if you can handle A2 milk.
>
> There are some good theoretical reasons why people who have Crohn's or similar syndromes may be able to digest A2 milk. The reason is that it contains no A1 beta-casein (which is present in so called 'normal' milk), which breaks down to form a peptide beta casomorphin7, and which causes particular problems for people who have an impaired digestive system.
>
> No guarantees but you may be pleasantly surprised. There are no scientific trials but quite a lot of anecdotal evidence from users, backed up by the theoretical evidence ...

I concluded by explaining where it could be bought in Christchurch. Claire replied that she would give it a try and let me know how it affected her.

I heard nothing for about five weeks. Then in March 2005, while overseas I received the following response: 'I have been having A2 milk for about a month now, every morning on my cereal. There have been no adverse affects – which is great. I will be telling others at my support group.'

Some weeks later I went to have a talk with Claire. She explained in more detail what she could eat and what she could not. I had been surprised to read in her email that she was putting the milk on cereal, as my understanding was that cereals were off the menu because of their laxative effects. Claire explained to me that she could eat simple cereals but not muesli bars, apart from one particular variety which she always carried in her bag. Knowing that muesli bars are typically held together with casein (or milk-protein concentrate, which is full of casein) I was intrigued and asked her to show me the one type of bar she could eat. Much to my interest, this particular bar used whey protein instead of casein. It just happened to be the only muesli bar I could find on the market that was free of casein and hence also free of the BCM7-forming A1 beta-casein. So it all fitted together. Subsequently I have asked Claire several times how she is going with the A2 milk and she says 'great'. I have also asked her whether she is still sure she can't drink ordinary milk. With a little smile, she replied that ordinary milk leads to a digestive explosion within half an hour.

The second anecdote is about an Australian friend of mine whose daughter suffers from coeliac disease. This is an intestinal disease caused by sensitivity to the gluten in wheat, barley and rye. It destroys the villi (tiny fingerlike protruberances in the wall of the small intestine) and so causes poor nutrient absorption. Untreated sufferers have great problems with diarrhoea and general wasting. If untreated they also have high rates of intestinal cancers and also increased risk of mental illness. (I will return to this last issue later in this chapter). Typically, newly diagnosed coeliac sufferers cannot digest milk products, but once they get off the gluten and the small intestine repairs itself they are once again able to digest milk (but not gluten-containing products). However, in the case of my friend's daughter, she is not only a coeliac but also has mild allergies and intolerance to milk, with symptoms including sinus conditions, asthma and intestinal bloating. So I suggested trying A2 milk, on the basis that it couldn't do any harm and might do some good. My friend reports back to me periodically that his daughter (and the rest of the family) now drink A2 milk, and do so without problems.

It is interesting to consider why some people can digest goats' milk but not cows' milk. Both types are broadly similar in relation to their protein types and lactose content. But goats' milk is A2 milk. There is also evidence from Israel that some people who are allergic to cows' milk can drink camels' milk, which also happens to be A2.[2] The authors of that study have identified BCM7 as a possible explanation.

What we don't know is the extent to which we can generalise from all of this anecdotal information about allergy and intolerance. Not everyone is going to be able to digest A2 milk: people who have a genuine lactose intolerance are still going to have a problem. And there are definitely other potential problems related to other proteins in both ordinary and A2 milk. For example, there are a few people (fortunately very few) who have extreme reactions to milk, including anaphylactic shock. These people need to avoid all milk products – whether from ordinary cows, A2 cows or goats. Some babies are even allergic to breast milk.

In response to the Australian media claims from consumers, a group of South Australian medics from AllergySA wrote a letter to the *Medical Journal of Australia* in 2004 outlining some tests they had done on 11 milk-allergic children.[3] They skin-pricked the children with both ordinary and A2 milk and measured the allergic reaction of the skin by the size of the weal that formed. They found no statistically significant differences between the reactions to the two types of milk. I have two comments on this. The first is that 'many' (it was not stated how many) of these children had previously suffered 'severe allergic reactions' to milk. These are clearly the type of children who should not be exposed to any dairy products except under close medical supervision. The second point is that these children didn't actually drink either the ordinary or the A2 milk (because of their history of severe reactions). BCM7 is only released when milk is digested, so it is highly doubtful that any effect it might have would show up in a skin test.

There is not a lot more to say about BCM7 and milk intolerance or allergies. In contrast to previous chapters that have focused on evidence published in scientific journals, so far in this chapter I have focused mainly on consumer reactions. Scientists tend to downplay such reports as anecdotal, but that does not mean that they should be ignored. What we now need is some good double-blind trials of people who have been identified as either milk-intolerant (e.g. they get bloating and diarrhoea) or mildly milk-allergic (e.g. who suffer from sinus, asthma or hives but are not at risk of anaphylactic shock). It should not be a hard trial to do, particularly for diarrhoea. It would certainly be much easier than trials relating to the effect of BCM7 on heart disease, Type 1 diabetes or autism. This would be a great investigation for a gastroenterologist.

One recent piece of the puzzle is a 2006 paper on the effect of BCM7 on the production of mucus.[4] There has been a widespread belief amongst the general public, going back at least 100 years, that milk consumption can cause excessive production of mucus in the nasal passages and throat. Indeed a Google search on 'mucus' and 'milk' brings up more than a million website references for the combined terms. However, the medical literature is widely sceptical about the mucus/milk relationship. The accepted view has been that it is a myth, because science had been unable to show a mucogenic effect. However, French and Spanish scientists have now shown, using mucus-producing intestinal tissues removed from humans, that BCM7 does indeed stimulate secretion of mucin (the proteins in mucus). They were able to show an increase of 69% over the controls. And they were able to demonstrate by use of the opioid antagonist cyprodyme that it was an opioid effect. So this would be consistent with producing mucus that was thicker and more sticky in the throat – exactly what many people claim as their symptoms.

In the second part of this chapter the focus shifts to a range of auto-immune diseases, most of which seem to be linked to leaky guts. In simple terms, auto-immune diseases can be thought of as diseases where the body has an allergy to itself. Instead of sending out antibodies to attack the foreign invaders, it somehow manages to get confused and damage itself. The question is: to what extent is the milk devil implicated?

With any of these auto-immune diseases, if there is a link to A1 beta-casein then there is likely to be a common factor – a leaky gut, which allows protein fragments (peptides) to enter the bloodstream and cause mayhem. The body reacts not only by forming antibodies to attack these peptides, but can also get fooled into attacking similar sequences of amino acids. The fundamental cause of leaky gut may itself be an auto-immune response to some virus, toxin, bacteria or food protein. Indeed it may be caused by any one of a great range of physiological stresses. The gut permeability may be either temporary or permanent.

In some cases the fundamental cause of a leaky gut may be linked to milk, but in most cases it probably won't be. The milk devil, BCM7, gets into the bloodstream as an outcome, without being the original causative agent. But once there, the BCM7 can roam widely. So once again, it seems to be a case of something else loading the gun and the milk devil pulling the trigger.

Coeliac disease

Coeliac disease is generally accepted as being an auto-immune disease. For a long time it was believed that people of northern European ethnicity were genetically more prone to this disease than other ethnic groups. However, people from other regions of the world, including the Middle East, northern Africa and India are now being increasingly diagnosed with this disease, and at similar incidence levels to northern Europe.[5]

I explained earlier in this chapter that coeliac disease occurs when the small intestine (usually but not necessarily the upper part) is damaged by a reaction to gluten. The small intestine is lined by villi, tiny finger-like structures which protrude from the wall of the intestine. These in turn have microvilli attached to them. The villi and microvilli increase the absorptive area of the small intestine, and produce and carry enzymes that help break down food. Once damage occurs, apparently through an auto-immune response, the digestive process is interfered with. In part this is because there is now a shortage of enzymes, and in part it is because the absorptive area is reduced. Also, the damaged lining may no longer be impervious to peptides from gluten, milk or indeed other protein sources. So coeliac sufferers are highly likely to have a leaky gut.

Untreated coeliacs are also intolerant of milk. This makes sense because the villi are no longer producing the lactase to digest the lactose sugar. But once gluten is removed from the diet, and the intestine wall has had time for self-repair, people with coeliac disease can typically once again digest milk.

However, there is an intriguing issue. It is that sufferers from coeliac disease are not always diagnosed, and if diagnosis does occur it is often only belatedly. When coeliac sufferers stop eating gluten products they often talk of the 'lifting of a mental fog'. Also, a recent Danish study published in the *British Medical Journal* found the risk factor for schizophrenia among people with coeliac disease to be 3.2 times higher than in the general population.[6] Indeed there seems to be general acceptance that coeliac sufferers are considerably more likely than the general population to suffer from neurological conditions. This is particularly the case if they are either undiagnosed (a common problem, especially in the early stages) or insufficiently disciplined to adhere to a gluten-free diet.

In the case of coeliac disease, no-one is suggesting that the disease itself is triggered by casomorphins from A1 beta-casein. We know that coeliac disease is caused by peptides in gluten. But once the intestine is damaged then the chances of the milk devil BCM7 slipping into the bloodstream are greatly enhanced. Also, Dr Sun and his colleagues from University of Florida have found that BCM7 passes through the blood/brain barrier much more easily and in a different way to the peptides from gluten, and the BCM7 attaches to 45 different parts of the brain.[7] To me, it seems to make sense as a simple matter of risk management that these people would be safer on A2 milk that does not release A1 beta-casein.

There is another piece of evidence that seems to confirm there is something going on in relation to coeliac disease and beta-casein. An

Italian group from the University of Rome found that coeliac patients had significantly higher levels of beta-casein antibodies than age-matched controls, and similar levels of these antibodies to people with Type 1 diabetes.[8] A p value of 0.02 for these data indicates the probability of getting this result by chance is only 2%. So we have to put this in the category of being an important signpost.

There is also a 1999 paper by Italian researchers in the journal *Gastroenterology* reporting that the longer coeliac sufferers remain exposed to gluten, the more likely they are to develop another auto-immune disorder.[9] On average, people with coeliac disease had a 14% chance of another auto-immune disease, compared to a 2.8% chance for age-matched controls. But among those who were not diagnosed until they were more than 10 years old, 24% had another auto-immune disease as well. Indeed coeliac disease seems to be associated with a great many neurological and developmental conditions.[10]

Crohn's disease and ulcerative colitis

These are distinct diseases, but are often grouped together as 'inflammatory bowel disease' or IBD. Crohn's disease is a patchy inflammation that can affect the full thickness of any part of the gastrointestinal tract. Ulcerative colitis affects only the colon, and only its inner lining. It is a continuous inflammation that starts near the anus and then works up through the colon. Both diseases are found mainly in northern Europe (particularly Scandinavia and Britain), North America, Australia, New Zealand and South Africa. The incidence of both diseases has increased greatly in the last 50 years. Sufferers sometimes need to have a section of their bowel surgically removed. Even without this surgery, these diseases impose a big constraint on normal living.

It is almost certain that the causes of Crohn's disease and ulcerative colitis are multi-factorial. Dr Richard Gearry has been undertaking an extensive survey of IBD sufferers in Christchurch, where I live, to try and identify risk factors. In April 2006, to a packed audience of more than 300 at an evening lecture at Christchurch Hospital, he presented his major findings. Presumably these findings will soon be available in a scientific journal.[11] He found that heredity was important and probably what primed the gun, but that it took one or possibly several external factors to pull the trigger. Exposure to animals and access to a vegetable garden as a child decreased the likelihood of getting the disease, and an urban upbringing increased the likelihood. This is consistent with the 'hygiene hypothesis': that as we decrease our exposure to germs in the environment, our body is increasingly likely to get fooled into attacking itself. It is as if the body *has* to have something to fight against, and if there is nothing better to do it will fight itself.

Another intriguing factor in both diseases is that breastfed babies are less likely to get them. It seems that breastfeeding has to occur for more than two months to provide the protective effect, and the risk declines the longer that breastfeeding is continued, up to and beyond 12 months. The confidence limits that Richard Gearry presented in his graphs indicated that the results were statistically significant, i.e. unlikely to be due to chance. I was initially sceptical about the accuracy of this information until one of Gearry's colleagues explained to me that most records in Plunket books are very well kept. Apparently very few mothers ever throw out their Plunket books!

There would seem to be two reasons why breastfeeding might help. The first is the presence of maternal antibodies in colostrum, which is produced in the breast milk in the first few days following birth. But that would hardly explain the decreasing incidence of Crohn's disease and ulcerative colitis for those people whose breastfeeding continued to three months, six months and beyond. The other alternative is that it is not just the protective effect of the breast milk, but the avoidance of formula milk derived from cows' milk. And if this is the case, then what could the milk component be?

Whatever the answer to the above question, what is known for sure is that a considerable proportion of Crohn's disease and ulcerative colitis sufferers are intolerant of ordinary milk. Unlike coeliac disease, where there is a logical reason why sufferers might be lactase deficient, and hence unable to digest lactose, there is no ready explanation here. This is particularly the case for ulcerative colitis, which is in a totally different part of the digestive system from where the villi are. There is also some evidence from Denmark that Crohn's and ulcerative colitis sufferers have an increased risk of schizophrenia.[12] These researchers found an increased risk of 40% for both diseases. In the case of ulcerative colitis the probability level was $p= 0.03$, which is statistically significant (only 3% likelihood of obtaining this result by chance). In the case of Crohn's, $p= 0.08$, which is not significant (because there is an 8% likelihood of getting such a result by chance) but this does not mean it is not real or unimportant. Rather, it means that there is too much variability in the data to exclude the possibility that it is a fluke. It would need to be confirmed through further studies and preferably with larger groups of people.

There is yet another piece of intriguing evidence relating to IBD. A paper published in the *Lancet* in 1995 gave evidence that these diseases were associated with lesions in the white matter of the brain, as measured by MRI scans.[13] Also, the previously mentioned Italian study, which found that coeliac sufferers had a much greater probability of having other auto-immune diseases, also found similar results for Crohn's disease.[14] They found that Crohn's sufferers were 4.6 times more likely than non-sufferers of Crohn's to also have another auto-immune disease.

Sudden infant death syndrome (SIDS)

In developed countries this is the most important cause of death in infants less than one year of age. These babies die unexpectedly and for no apparent reason. They are perfectly well when tucked up in their cots, and then they are found dead a few hours later.

There is clear evidence that there is no single cause. Rather, there are several and possibly many factors that can contribute to SIDS, and some others that are protective. A smoking environment is harmful. It is also important that babies should not be laid down to sleep on their stomachs. Breastfeeding appears to be strongly protective. Why should all this be so?

The link between SIDS and casomorphins that are derived from casein goes back to at least 1988. At that time a paper exploring this link was written by two American scientists from New York University Medical Centre.[15] Back then no-one understood that the important casomorphins (BCM7 and its derivatives such as BCM5) were released from A1 beta-casein and not A2 beta-casein. But the possibility that SIDS could be caused by respiratory depression from these opioids was already gaining attention.

Since then there have been several trials with young animals showing that injections of BCM7 cause breathing irregularities.[16] Also, it has been shown that young animals absorb BCM7 from the intestine much more readily than do adult animals. Recently, Dr Sun and colleagues have published a paper in the journal *Peptides*, setting out how they believe the SIDS response may be occurring.[17]

Multiple sclerosis

Multiple sclerosis, or MS, is one of the most puzzling of diseases. It is a classic auto-immune disease, caused by the body attacking the myelin sheath that surrounds nerves. The disease greatly affects mobility but tends to be spasmodic, with recurring attacks that usually get progressively worse. The generally accepted belief is that there is no cure. However, there is also an intriguing body of evidence that it can be treated by eliminating food proteins that have been relatively recently (over the last few thousand years) added to the human diet – in particular milk protein and gluten. The theory is that some people carry genes that make them more susceptible to these recent additions to the human diet. Some genes that increase susceptibility have even been identified. However, it is also very clear that there are environmental triggers. The challenge is to work out what these triggers are.

It has long been recognised that multiple sclerosis has something to do with where people live, particularly in the early part of their lives. People who live in high latitudes (away from the equator) are very much more likely to have the disease than people who live in low latitudes (near the equator). People who shift from low latitudes as adults retain the risk factor of their country of origin, but their children have the risk factor of the country of destination. This suggests that there is probably a long lag phase between when the environmental trigger is pulled and when the disease manifests itself. So what are the environmental factors that are linked to latitude?

Vitamin D has long been considered a potential factor. The major source of this vitamin is sunlight. People in high latitudes are exposed to less sunlight, particularly in winter. But it is easy to pick holes in the vitamin D theory. To start with, Japanese people living in Hawai'i have a three times higher incidence of multiple sclerosis than those living in Japan, although Hawai'i is closer to the equator. And there are plenty of other flaws in the theory. So the attention has turned back to food items as at least part of the trigger mechanism.

Ashton Embry is a Canadian who has played a key role in bringing together the disparate sources of information on the causes of multiple sclerosis. He has set up a charity (MS-direct) dedicated to finding the causes of multiple sclerosis. The charity searches out and also funds relevant studies. The charity has an excellent website: www.direct-ms.org.

Ashton Embry is himself the father of a son who developed multiple sclerosis. This is what caused him to become so interested in the disease.

Embry's own training was as a geologist searching for oil and minerals, not as a medical scientist. But as a research scientist he had been trained to seek out the most likely explanations from incomplete and sometimes apparently conflicting evidence. When evidence appears to conflict, a good starting point is to look at the starting assumptions, on the basis that if you don't ask the right questions you can't expect to find the right answers. Similarly, if there are two competing theories, a set of essential criteria needs to be developed against which they can be judged. These principles apply just as much in medicine as in geology.

When Embry found that his son had MS his immediate aim was to identify a life strategy that would at least slow down and preferably cure the disease. He soon worked out that a diet low in dairy products, cereal grains and legumes was the most promising approach. This is sometimes called the paleolithic approach because of its focus on foods that humans ate about 10,000 years ago, prior to the development of agriculture. Although the diet is highly restrictive, many people who follow it – including Embry's son – report long-term remission. This is in stark contrast to the apparent lack of similar reports from other approaches.

An epidemiological study by French researchers D. Malosse and colleagues linking multiple sclerosis to milk consumption was published in the journal *Neuroepidemiology* in 1992. It showed a strong correlation between milk intake and multiple sclerosis for 27 countries, and that this was statistically significant at $p< 0.001$ (less than 0.1% probability of obtaining such a result by chance). One of the weaknesses of this study was that it included a diverse range of countries with greatly different lifestyles. This increases the risk that the apparent correlations are non-causal. However, when I re-ran the data for 16 wealthy OECD countries there was still a statistically significant relationship.

Further attempts that I made to investigate these relationships, including the link to A1 beta-casein, were thwarted by data problems. Those problems went right back to the issue of getting good data on the prevalence (i.e. the level of the disease in the population) and the incidence (i.e. the rate at which new cases were appearing). With a disease such as Type 1 diabetes a single criterion for whether people have the disease is very simple: it is based on the need for insulin injections. But with multiple sclerosis the criteria are many, less clear and not necessarily applied consistently across international boundaries. Indeed, when I compared the various data on prevalence and incidence (both separately and together) I found considerable differences in the estimates within individual countries. My own analyses using published data showed that countries with high levels of multiple sclerosis also had high levels of Type 1 diabetes, high heart disease, and high intakes of milk. All of these relationships were statistically significant. But it was impossible to tease anything else out from the murky data relating to A1 beta-casein.

The idea that multiple sclerosis is linked to milk refuses to go away. A study in the *Lancet* back in 1974 may have been the first to make the link.[18] More recently, an American study linked multiple sclerosis in the USA to a diet low in fish and high in dairy products.[19]

In 2002 a study in the *Lancet* reported that in Sardinia, Italy, people with multiple sclerosis were three to five times more likely than their siblings to have Type 1 diabetes.[20] Also, having relatives with multiple sclerosis increased the risk of being diabetic by a factor of six. This article led to considerable comment, both in the *Lancet* and elsewhere, that the association of these two diseases was an 'unlikely alliance'. The reasoning was the conventional wisdom that some specific genes believed to increase the risk of multiple sclerosis were also believed to be protective against Type 1 diabetes. However, a group of American researchers led by Janice Dorman were sufficiently intrigued to go back and look at some peripheral data they had collected in another study looking at the clustering of Type 1 diabetes, auto-immune thyroid disease and rheumatoid arthritis.[21] First they 'pleaded guilty' that previously they had failed to look for a possible association between Type 1 diabetes and multiple sclerosis because they had assumed it would not exist. They found a 20-fold increase in the prevalence of multiple sclerosis among their Type 1 diabetic women and concluded that 'adult women with Type 1 diabetes are at an enormously increased risk of multiple sclerosis, and that the answer to questions about the clustering of these disorders is that they are [linked] together at last'.

This, of course, raises at least as many questions as it might answer. But it is fascinating that these two diseases seem to have common genetic risk factors and a common environmental risk factor in relation to milk. This is further supported by another paper by some of the authors of the Sardinian study, this time published in the journal *Human Molecular Genetics* in 2004, suggesting that there is indeed a common environmental factor linking to the genetic factor.[22]

There is further evidence linking these two diseases. Michael Dosch, Professor of Paediatrics and Immunology at the University of Toronto, led a team that has investigated similarities between the two diseases. The work has been published in the *Journal of Immunology* in 2001.[23] In a press release Michael Dosch said, 'Much to our surprise, we found immunologically Type 1 diabetes and multiple sclerosis are almost the same – in a test tube you can barely tell the two diseases apart.'

Also, Kalle Reichelt has recently turned his attention to multiple sclerosis and reports finding increased levels of IgA antibodies to gluten, gliadin and casein.[24] One can only wonder where this intriguing research will lead.

Parkinson's disease

This is a neuro-degenerative disorder which is poorly understood. It causes people to shake and to have difficulty transmitting instructions from the brain to the limbs. It is linked to the loss of dopamine-producing cells in the brain, and sometimes listed as an auto-immune disease. The cause is unknown. Pesticides are suspected in some cases. Caffeine appears to be protective, with one study finding non-coffee-drinkers five times more at risk than heavy coffee drinkers.[25] There are no good data on how the incidence of Parkinson's varies between countries or ethnic groups. Some countries such as China are widely believed to have a very low level and others such as Argentina apparently have a very high level. However, the statistics may not be reliable. The prevalence of Parkinson's is apparently increasing but this is probably only because average lifespan has increased. In general it is a disease of later life.

The most rigorous analyses of factors linked to Parkinson's disease have been undertaken by a team from the Harvard School of Public Health, led by Dr Alberto Ascherio. The team has numerous publications investigating a wide range of food and lifestyle factors.[26] Their initial key data sources were long-term studies of 50,000 male health professionals and 120,000 nurses, and more recently some 130,000 men and women from the American Cancer Society's long-term Cancer Prevention Study. They have found strong supportive evidence that both caffeine and smoking are protective. No, that is not a misprint! Non-smokers are considerably more likely to get Parkinson's than are smokers.

The reason for this is far from clear. But one possibility is what is called 'reverse causality': that lack of dopamine (which leads to Parkinson's) is also associated with non-risk-taking personality types who are less likely to smoke. But this is just a hypothesis: we simply don't know. However, the important finding for the issues discussed in this book is that there is one food item that Dr Ascherio and colleagues keep finding associated with Parkinson's disease: milk. And it is the *only* food type that appears to be a risk factor clearly associated with Parkinson's. A large-scale study of Japanese-American men in Honolulu also found similar results.

Dr Ascherio's team has attempted to identify what the component in milk might be that could be causing the problem. The researchers think it is unlikely to be fat because when they look at total fat in the diet the correlation is less strong. Also, they believe for the same reasons that it is unlikely to be calcium or total protein intake. So what is the special component in milk that is causing the problem? Dr Ascherio's team have looked at reverse causality (i.e. the idea that people drink more milk because they have low dopamine levels) but found no support for this. They have also looked at whether the cause might be pesticides in the milk. This is a possibility, particularly for the Honolulu study, because it is well documented that in 1981/82 there was heptachlor contamination of milk in some parts of Hawai'i from cows eating contaminated pineapple leaves. But overall, they suggest that the milk in American diets is unlikely to be a major source of ingested pesticides. So they keep coming back to the idea that there is something in milk that is causing a problem but it is unrelated to the calcium level, or the fat content, or to the total level of protein.

I have written to Dr Ascherio and suggested that they might like to look at BCM7. But once again, it will not be an easy task to prove this in scientifically controlled diets. Perhaps it needs a different team, such as that led by Dr Sun, to explore what happens to dopamine-producing cells when BCM7 is injected into animals. And perhaps it needs a team of immunologists to explore whether or not there are beta-casein antibodies in Parkinson's sufferers. There is plenty of work to do!

The big picture

Once again, readers can now use the evidence to draw their own conclusions. In the case of milk intolerance and allergy, it seems likely that A1 beta-casein, and the milk devil BCM7 that is derived from it, are indeed implicated. Is it likely that so many consumers could all be wrong, particularly when the symptoms, such as diarrhoea, are well defined? Also, the story is totally consistent with what we know of the pharmacology and biochemistry of BCM7.

In the case of the auto-immune diseases discussed in this chapter, the story is somewhat more murky and speculative. What we do know for sure is that for each disease there is one or more environmental trigger. We also know that milk keeps coming up as a prime candidate. If milk contains the cause then it almost certainly has to be one or more bio-active proteins in the milk. It is also likely that opioids are involved. It is hard to go past BCM7 as a likely candidate.

We also need to remember that the auto-immune story is very much a work in progress. Most of the references listed for this section have only been published since 2000. I will be watching with great interest over the next few years as the mists slowly disperse and a much clearer picture emerges. Undoubtedly there will be false leads, and the answers will be complex. It seems to me that BCM7 is leaving enough tell-tale signs that it is eventually going to be unmasked as a villain. Surely it would be better that our milk was free of this devil.

In the next chapter I will therefore discuss how we can, through selective breeding, eliminate A1 beta-casein from milk. But of course that will only happen if consumers make it clear to our dairy industry that this is what they want to happen.

NOTES

1 See American Autoimmune Related Diseases Association website www.aarda.org. Accessed 29 April 2007.

2 See Shabo *et al* (2005) in Allergies, Intolerance and Auto-immune Conditions section of Bibliography.

3 See Smith *et al* (2004) in Allergies, Intolerance and Auto-immune Conditions section of Bibliography.

4 See Zoghbi *et al* (2006) in Allergies, Intolerance and Auto-immune Conditions section of Bibliography.

5 See Malekzadeh *et al* (2005) in Allergies, Intolerance and Auto-immune Conditions section of Bibliography

6 See Eaton *et al* (2004) in Allergies, Intolerance and Auto-immune Conditions section of Bibliography.

7 See Sun *et al* (1999) and Sun and Cade (2003), both in Autism and Schizophrenia section of Bibliography.

8 See Monetini *et al* (2002) in Allergies, Intolerance and Auto-immune Conditions section of Bibliography.

9 See Ventura *et al* (1999) in Allergies, Intolerance and Auto-immune Conditions section of Bibliography.

10 See Bushara (2005) in Allergies, Intolerance and Auto-immune Conditions section of Bibliography.

11 Some aspects of the study concerning incidence levels but not the correlations with other factors were published in late 2006. See Geary *et al* (2006) in Allergies, Intolerance and Auto-immune Conditions section of Bibliography.

12 See Eaton *et al* (2004) in Allergies, Intolerance and Auto-immune Conditions section of Bibliography.

13 See Geissler *et al* (1995) in Allergies, Intolerance and Auto-immune Conditions section of Bibliography. There remains debate about the medical implications of these lesions.

14 See Ventura *et al* (1999) in Allergies, Intolerance and Auto-immune Conditions section of Bibliography.

15 See Ramabadran and Bansinath (1988) in Milk and Casomorphins section of Bibliography.

16 See Hedner and Hedner (1987) and Taira *et al* (1990) in Milk and Casomorphins section of Bibliography.

17 See Sun *et al* (2003) in Milk and Casomorphins section of Bibliography.

18 See Agranoff and Goldberg (1974) in Allergies, Intolerance and Auto-immune Conditions section of Bibliography.

19 See Lauer (1994) in Allergies, Intolerance and Auto-immune Conditions section of Bibliography.

20 See Marrosu *et al* (2002) in Allergies, Intolerance and Auto-immune Conditions section of Bibliography.

21 See Dorman *et al* (2003) in Allergies, Intolerance and Auto-immune Conditions section of Bibliography.

22 See Marrosu *et al* (2004) in Allergies, Intolerance and Auto-immune Conditions section of Bibliography.

23 See Winer *et al* (2001) in Allergies, Intolerance and Auto-immune Conditions section of Bibliography.

24 See Reichelt and Jensen (2004) in Allergies, Intolerance and Auto-immune Conditions section of Bibliography.

25 See Ross *et al* (2000) in Allergies, Intolerance and Auto-immune Conditions section of Bibliography.

26 Their 2007 publication in the *American Journal of Epidemiology* is particularly important. See Chen *et al* (2007) in Allergies, Intolerance and Auto-immune Conditions section of Bibliography.

CHAPTER TEN

BREEDING A2 COWS

There is nothing difficult about breeding a herd of A2 cows. Farmers merely need to use either A2 bulls, or semen that is known to come from A2 bulls. Then it is simply a case of waiting for nature to take its course. However there are a number of strategies that farmers can use to speed up the rate of change. One of these is to genetically test the cows and then cull selectively. Another is to genetically test all calves. A third is to increase the rate at which young cows, called heifers, are brought into the herd. And of course it also depends on the initial level of the A2 allele within a herd.

Because of all the variables involved I am always cautious about generalisations stating how long it will take to convert a herd. But with a concerted effort it is possible to convert most herds to pure A2 within about 10 years, and in some situations, less.

Some simple genetics

If farmers want to make rapid progress towards achieving an A2 herd then an understanding of simple animal genetics is helpful.

The A1/A2 status of a cow is determined by a pair of genes on the sixth chromosome. Cows and bulls each carry two copies of this gene. Also, there are two major alleles (variants) of the gene – the A1 and A2 beta-casein alleles. (Actually there are at least eight variants of the gene, but the remainder are subsets of the A1 and A2 variants and do not need to be considered separately.)

Because a cow carries two copies of the gene, she can carry either two copies of the A2 allele, two copies of the A1 allele, or one copy of each. The three states are referred to as homozygous A2A2, homozygous A1A1, and heterozygous A1A2.

Where both alleles occur together (A1A2) neither is dominant over the other. Instead, they are co-dominant, i.e. additive in their effect. Therefore an A1A2 cow will produce both A1 beta-casein and A2 beta-casein in equal amounts in her milk. A cow that is A2A2 will only produce A2 beta-casein and a cow that is A1A1 will only produce A1 beta-casein.

The A1 mutation occurred thousands of years ago in some early European cattle, so only European cattle produce milk containing A1 beta-casein. However, European bloodlines exist in many cattle that look as if they are either African or Asian. Therefore no animal can be assumed from its outward appearance to be A2A2. For example, the dominant tropical beef breed of cattle in Brazil is the Nelore. These cattle, which are also crossbred in the tropical north with European breeds for milking purposes, are usually described as being a *Bos indicus* breed, i.e. of Asian origin. However, Brazilian colleagues tell me that the so-called 'pure' Nelore carry the A1 allele at a level of about 7%, which probably means that they carry about 15% European ancestry. The milking crossbreds will carry the A1 allele at a considerably higher level than this, but still much lower than in pure European breeds.

The dairy industries of most developed countries are based on European breeds. As a very broad generalisation, herds based on the Northern European black-and-white breeds such as Holstein/Friesian will typically carry the A1 and A2 alleles at about equal levels. The southern European breeds and the Jersey are likely to carry the A1 allele at about 35%. There are also plenty of exceptions. For example the European Guernsey breed appears to be less than 10% A1 and the Scottish Ayrshire breed appears to be well over 50%.

Particularly important is the fact that individual herds may carry an incidence of the A1 allele that is quite different to the average for that breed. If a farmer has used semen from a small number of bulls then it is very easy to end up by chance with a level that is either considerably higher or considerably lower than the average.

Taking a typical black-and-white herd of cows, i.e. of Holstein/Friesian origin, then perhaps 25% might be A2A2, 50% A1A2, and 25% A1A1. This combination would produce milk with a 50:50 ratio of A1 to A2 beta-casein.

If a cow is A2A2 then it is guaranteed to pass on the A2 allele to its progeny. Similarly, if a cow is A1A1 it is guaranteed to pass on a copy of the A1 allele to its progeny. But if a cow is A1A2 it may pass on either the A1 or the A2 allele, with a 50% probability for each.

Once we understand the principle that a newly conceived calf has two copies of the gene – one from the cow and one from the bull – it is straightforward to work out what will happen if an A2A2 bull is mated to the abovementioned cows :

- If an A2A2 bull is mated to an A2A2 cow then all the progeny will be A2A2.
- If an A2A2 bull is mated to a cow that is A1A2, then half the progeny will be A2A2 and the other half will be A1A2.
- If a bull that is A2A2 is mated to a cow that is A1A1, then all the progeny will be A1A2.

Three further pieces of information are needed to work out how fast the A1/A2 beta-casein status of a herd can be changed. The first is the gestation period, i.e. the period of pregnancy. This is about 282 days plus or minus a few days depending on the breed and individual characteristics of both the cow and the sire to which she is mated. The second piece of information is the age at which a young cow will first calve and therefore start producing milk. On most modern dairy farms this is two years. The third piece of information is the herd replacement rate. In New Zealand and Australia this is typically about 20% but in many European and American herds it is about 35%. With cows calving every year, in theory it should be mathematically possible, with a 50:50 ratio of male and female calves, to replace 50% of the cows each year. In practice this never happens. For example some cows fail to get in calf, some calves are either born dead or die as young calves, and some die before reaching mature age. In practice the maximum replacement rate is likely to be about 40%.

Taking together the information about gestation and age of first calving, we can see that it will be nearly three years after a decision is made to mate exclusively with A2A2 bulls before there is any effect on the A1/A2 composition of the milk produced by that herd. From then on, reasonably rapid progress can be made depending on the herd replacement rate.

- If 20% of the herd is replaced each year, and starting with an assumed 50% A2 content of the milk, then the level of A2 will increase by about 5% each year, i.e. increasing to 55% in the fourth year and 60% in the fifth year and so on.
- If 20% of the herd is replaced each year but the initial A2 content of the milk is only 20% then this can be increased each year by

about 8%, i.e. reaching about 28% in the fourth year and 36% in the fifth year.

- If the initial A2 content of the milk is 50% but there is a 35% herd replacement rate then the A2 content would increase to about 58% in the fourth year and 67% in the fifth year.

These rates of improvement are based on using A2 semen but not testing the cows or progeny. I call this the 'passive approach' to breeding A2 cows. Unfortunately, the rate of improvement with this approach will slow down with each successive generation of cows. So starting with a herd at 50% level of the A2 allele, and with a cow replacement rate of 20% per annum, there will have been:

- no improvement in the first three years
- an increase in the A2 content of the milk to about 75% by year 8
- an increase in the A2 content of the milk to about 87% by year 13
- an increase in the A2 content of the milk to about 94% by year 18.

This relationship is what mathematicians call 'asymptotic'. It means that the herd will eventually get close to pure but will never be totally pure. To get a totally pure herd each cow must be individually tested. And the earlier this occurs then the faster the whole process can become, first by culling A1A1 cows and then A1A2 cows, and second by better calf selection decisions.

Another factor that can speed up the conversion to A2 is by selecting the calves of heifers (young cows) that are calving for the first time and which are themselves A2A2. This might seem obvious but in practice many farmers do not keep the calves from first-calving cows. There are two reasons for this.

The first reason is that if 15-month heifers are to be artificially mated then they need to be yarded regularly to monitor their ovulation status, whereas milking cows are already being yarded daily for milking. Often the young stock are agisted out on another property. So on a busy farm it can be easier letting the replacement livestock 'go back to nature' and let a bull work out these matters for himself. The bull is unlikely to be of equivalent genetic merit to the top bulls used in the artificial insemination programme, and so these progeny are not kept.

The second reason is that first-calving heifers sometimes have difficulty calving. Hence, they are sometimes mated to bulls selected according to their ability to sire small calves, rather than bulls that will produce the top milk-producing progeny. Despite these issues, there is no technical reason why heifers cannot be artificially inseminated just like the older cows, and in New Zealand about 20% of farmers do this.

Because of the large number of variables involved there is no simple figure for the number of years it will take to convert a herd from its existing state to pure A2. If people want a 'ballpark' figure I usually say ten years for a typical herd in Europe, North America, South America, New Zealand and Australia. Some farmers will be able to complete the conversion by the seventh year if they do everything possible to speed up the process. And of course an individual farmer can speed things up even further by purchasing A2 cows from other farmers. But at the national level the purchasing option is what is called a 'zero-sum' gain. In other words it is only through breeding, and not through buying and selling between farmers, that the national herd can change its overall status.

In some other parts of the world, a pure A2 herd can be produced more quickly than this. In countries like India many of the local herds are probably already close to pure A2. However, even in India there will have been some infusion of European cattle genes, and in the cooler parts of India there may be quite a high level of European cattle genes, particularly in the larger commercial herds.

Testing cows and bulls

It is easy to test the status of cows by typing the DNA, using several hairs plucked from the tail. The test is currently available in New Zealand, Australia and the USA. It can readily be made available elsewhere. The patent is held by A2 Corporation in New Zealand but the test can easily be done by arrangement in laboratories outside New Zealand. Many farmers are already DNA-testing cows and calves for other purposes, so adding in the A2 test is straightforward.

Currently, farmers in many countries face constraints in getting semen that is guaranteed to be A2. This is simply because most farmers in these countries know nothing about the issue and have not demanded it. Once a few farmers say they want A2 semen the marketing companies will soon test their bulls and provide the information to their clients. Both of the major New Zealand companies market dairy semen all over the world, and I know of a farmer in Uruguay, for example, who is purchasing A2 semen from New Zealand.

For New Zealand farmers there is already no problem in purchasing A2 semen. The two major companies selling dairy semen, which between them have well over 95% of the market, have all of their New Zealand-based bulls catalogued by their A1/A2 status. However, there is no other country where this is done routinely. There is an irony here, in that the mainstream New Zealand dairy industry has been very 'upfront' in arguing against A2 milk. The rest of the world has to a large extent gone along with this perspective, and assumed that the Kiwis must know what they are doing. So these other countries have not bothered to set up testing of their own bulls in the way that New Zealand has.

In theory, there should be no need to test the progeny of A2A2 cows mated with A2A2 semen. Scientific logic says that the progeny must also be A2A2. There is only one problem: when several cows calve in a paddock overnight both cows and dairy farmers sometimes get confused as to which calf belongs to which cow. Genetic testing of herds in New Zealand indicates that there is about a 15% mistake rate. This is much less likely to be an issue for those European and American herds that calve indoors, often in separate cubicles.

The costs of using A2 semen

There are two types of cost that need to be considered. The first is the cash cost. The second is the reduced breeding options that farmers face through not being able to use semen from A1 bulls of otherwise high genetic merit.

For farmers to begin the process by using A2 semen involves very little cash cost. At present there is no market premium for A2 semen, although that may change in future. Alternatively viewed, in future A1 semen may sell at a discounted price.

The biggest potential cost of using A2 semen is that it could, at least in theory, restrict the feasible rate of herd improvement for other characteristics that farmers considered important. The reason for this is the well-known principle that the more factors you select for, the less progress is possible in relation to any individual factor. This principle is particularly important if the factor being selected for is influenced by multiple genes. In this regard it is fortunate that the A1/A2 beta-casein status is determined by only one gene, but this fact does not totally avoid the problem.

Peter Gatley, the General Manager Genetics for New Zealand's Livestock Improvement Corporation (LIC), writing in a letter to the *New Zealand Farmers Weekly* in May 2004, said that if only A2A2 bulls were used then 'current calculations indicate a five point drop in Breeding

Worth which translates into a cost of [NZ]$15 million'. This 'breeding worth' calculation measures the loss as a capital value. In proportion to the total industry investment of about NZ$40 billion this seems rather small. It is less than a third the value of one day's production of milk.

In practice even this might be an overestimate. In New Zealand we are finding that the majority of the top bulls (as determined by production traits) also happen to be A2A2. Remarkably, whereas the national cow herd is believed to contain the A1 and A2 alleles in the ratio of about 50:50, with about 25% of the cows A2A2, the national ranking list of top dairy bulls has an A2:A1 allele ratio of about 70:30 or even higher, and with more than half the top bulls being A2A2. The exact figure fluctuates somewhat as new bulls enter and old bulls exit the scheme. In other words, if farmers select their bull semen based on economically important criteria as measured in the national herd recording scheme, then they will significantly increase the level of the A2 allele without even trying. There has also been a recent published research paper showing that on average New Zealand A2 cows are higher-producing than New Zealand A1 cows.[1]

Whether this situation also applies in other countries is totally unknown, for the simple reason that their bulls and cows have not been tested. It may simply be a chance relationship that applies only to the New Zealand herd. Indeed this is highly likely, because the breeding criteria used in New Zealand's grass-fed system for production of protein and milkfat are different from those used in most other countries, where the emphasis is typically on milk volume produced from concentrates. Given that the A1 allele has survived for thousands of years it would be surprising if, across the world, it were to suddenly decline markedly without purposeful action by farmers.

The irony of this situation is obvious. Here is the New Zealand industry claiming that A1/A2 is a non-issue, yet the industry is drifting by accident towards A2. And consequently all of this is occurring with minimal publicity.

Several people have said to me that this looks too good to be true. It must be a conspiracy, they say. I always assure them this is extremely unlikely. I have no reason to question the integrity of the national bull ranking scheme, and indeed I believe it is inconceivable that there is any tampering with the results. To do so would be very silly and impossible to hide. It would be inevitable that someone would 'spill the beans'.

In any case, I believe the people who administer the scheme (and with whom I correspond regularly regarding professional matters unrelated to A2) are of unquestionable integrity. The facts are simply that in New Zealand at the moment, the progeny of the top A2 bulls are scoring particularly well for key production traits such as producing lots of protein relative to their size.

However, what is also notable is that in 2006 the New Zealand 'Premium Sires' scheme operated by LIC (previously known as Livestock Improvement Corporation) appeared to have an even higher ratio of A2 to A1 bulls than would be expected from the animal rankings. This 'Premium Sires' scheme is also known as 'bull of the day' and is used by more than half of New Zealand's dairy farmers. Essentially, the artificial insemination technician visits the farms in his or her 'round' each day carrying fresh semen from two high-ranking bulls for each breed. For each cow, semen from the first bull of the appropriate breed is used unless the cow is closely related to that bull, in which case semen from the back-up bull is used. It is notable that in 2006 there were several very good bulls that LIC had access to, that happened to be A1A2, that were omitted from the team of 'Premium Sires'. Whether this omission related to the A1 status or something else I cannot judge. However, one person who almost certainly would be in a position to know has said to me that I should not assume that it is random. Regardless, it is going to impact eventually on the overall ratio of the A2 allele in the New Zealand herd. For the 2007 season I have analysed the overall A2 level of the Premium Sires team as being 78%, which is consistent with the national bull ranking data for 2007.

Should farmers convert their herds to A2?

A small number of farmers in New Zealand, Australia, and now the USA have already converted their herds to A2. Those who have completed the process have typically done so because they have contracts to supply A2 milk for which they receive a premium price. To get rapidly to this pure status they have had to test their cows, and then typically purchase and test additional cows to get sufficient numbers. Some farmers have sufficient cows to run two separate herds, one being pure A2 and the other containing the A1A1 and A1A2 cows whose milk is being sold into the ordinary milk market.

Most dairy farmers are not currently being offered a contract for A2 milk. For these farmers the key question is whether they should start the conversion process now, knowing that it will take quite a few years to complete.

Essentially, it is a risk-management decision. Farmers have to look at the cost of conversion versus their estimate of what the A2 premium (or A1 discount) might be at some time in the future. They also have to weigh up the potential cost of converting their herd and there being no premium/discount, against the loss that might be incurred if there is a premium for A2 (or a discounted price for A1) and they have failed to convert.

Currently in New Zealand there are about 500 dairy farmers who are quietly converting their herds to A2 as a risk-management strategy. They are not necessarily convinced that they will gain a benefit, but they want to ensure that they do not end up getting a discount that might threaten their whole business. In most cases they have been taking the passive approach of using A2 semen but not testing their cows. Their rationale is that if a premium/discount does occur then at that stage they will test their cows and rapidly finish the conversion process.

The estimate of 500 converting farmers comes from a random survey in 2005 of 2000 dairy farmers undertaken by a postgraduate student at Lincoln University under my supervision. The purpose of the survey was to identify the breeding attributes that farmers want the artificial insemination companies to focus on, and about 4% of respondents said that they were already exclusively using A2 semen. If applied to the national herd this would mean about 500 farms. One of the two major breeding companies (Ambreed) has told me that about 10% of their clients are purposely using only A2 semen, but it is likely that this firm is not typical of the overall market.

What is clear, however, is that most New Zealand farmers continue to do nothing about A2. They are working on the premise that as their processing and marketing co-operative, Fonterra, has been telling them that A2 is a non-issue, they don't need to do anything about it.

In other countries almost no farmers have been breeding for A2. The reason is simply that until now they, like nearly all consumers, have known nothing about the issue.

NOTES

1 See Morris *et al* (2005) in Cattle Genetics section of Bibliography.

CHAPTER ELEVEN

THE FOOD SAFETY GAME

There was immediate consternation in the New Zealand Food Safety Authority (NZFSA) following publication of the Laugesen and Elliott paper in the *NZ Medical Journal* of January 2003. Within days the NZFSA issued a press release headed 'Milk Still Part of Balanced Diet'.

The press release reported factually that Laugesen and Elliott

> have found a significant correlation between the amount of A1 beta-casein and milk protein consumed in a country and the national rate of coronary heart disease. They also found a similar correlation between A1 beta-casein consumption and the rate of childhood type-1 diabetes ...
>
> The Ministry of Health supports the NZFSA's view that the evidence is not strong enough to change the health messages around milk or to require any special labelling on milk or milk product ... milk is nutritious and beneficial and should remain part of a balanced diet.

The NZFSA is a government organisation with multiple roles which may at times be conflicting. According to the home page of the NZFSA website as of May 2007 (www.nzfsa.govt.nz) it 'protects and promotes public health and safety', and 'facilitates access to markets for New Zealand food and food products'. So it both monitors and supports the food industry.

The NZFSA also works very closely with the Food Standards Authority of Australia and New Zealand, which is responsible for consistent labelling of food in both countries. Therefore, if the NZFSA decided that there were food-safety issues surrounding milk there would be implications for both countries.

Very soon after the release of the Laugesen and Elliott paper the NZFSA decided that it needed to hold an inquiry into the issues surrounding A1 and A2 milk. The reasoning behind the decision is a matter of conjecture, but as we will see in the next few pages, a reasonable interpretation could be that the NZFSA wanted to 'put a lid' on the matter as quickly as possible. At this time Fonterra and A2 Corporation were fighting each other in court, with A2 Corporation claiming that ordinary milk should carry a health warning. There was considerable concern that the A1/A2 issue had potential to damage the New Zealand dairy industry.

The following information about the way NZFSA went about setting up and influencing the inquiry comes from information obtained from the NZFSA itself using the disclosure powers of the Official Information Act 1982. Anybody can make a request for release of relevant official documents. The information reported here was obtained in March 2004 by Nigel Stirling, who was Editor of the *New Zealand Farmers' Weekly*. At the time I was writing some articles for that magazine about A2 milk and Nigel forwarded this information to me.

Unfortunately the NZFSA deleted some paragraphs and sections of paragraphs from the released documents. These were deemed confidential, mainly relating to specific comments about individuals. However, there was enough information remaining to tell an interesting story as to how the NZFSA works, and how it 'manages' information.

The correspondence released by the NZFSA shows that by 14 March 2003 it was well advanced in negotiations with Professor Boyd Swinburn from Deakin University in Australia, who was a former Medical Director of the National Heart Foundation of New Zealand, for him to undertake a review of the available information relating to A1 and A2 milk. However, A2 Corporation apparently knew nothing about this until Chief Executive Officer Dr Corran McLachlan read it in the *New Zealand Herald* towards the end of April. A transcript of a radio interview from the last week of April indicates that McLachlan was furious. He accused the NZFSA of 'not acting with a straight bat', and showing 'partisanship' in their choice of the reviewer. McLachlan was incensed because Swinburn was a former colleague of Bob Elliott at Auckland University and had just a few weeks previously described Elliott on the Australian television programme 'White Mischief' as a 'maverick'. It did seem, at least on the surface, that there might be some question as to his independence.

Correspondence to Boyd Swinburn from NZFSA's Policy Director,

Carole Inkster, is enlightening. In early April she wrote: 'we have had virtually no coverage of the A1/A2 milk issue here since the 4 Corners telecast in Aus earlier this week – which is quite a relief for us but I think perhaps a temporary reprieve.'

Later in April she responded to a question from Boyd Swinburn as to whether he should discuss the 'precautionary principle'. She wrote:

> In relation to discussion of the precautionary principle our preference would be not to discuss it as a precautionary principle – this term has all sorts of baggage associated with it (especially European baggage) and our preference is to refer to the way we treat uncertainty in scientific assessments and exercise caution in reaching risk management based positions. Happy to expand further on this if that would be useful.

And then in late May, when they were still finalising the terms of reference for the study (although she was expecting a draft of Boyd Swinburn's report only three days later), Inkster said she hoped to 'go out (trickle out) with a summary of the terms of reference'.[1]

The 'precautionary principle' is a basic principle used in matters where there are risks associated with a particular course of action or lack of action. It recognises that it could be disastrous to wait for final proof. An example is global warning. There is no absolute proof that man-made climate change is occurring on our planet, but there is some very powerful evidence for it. Actions that various governments and other groups are taking to mitigate the effects of climate change are based not on proof, but on the precautionary principle. In fact it is arguably exactly the reverse of what Carole Inkster of NZFSA seemed to be advocating in relation to exercising caution in reaching risk management based positions.

Boyd Swinburn also wrote a number of emails back to Carole Inkster at NZFSA reporting on progress. Initially he advised that he thought it would only be about a four-day job, and that his approach was to do a search of computer databases to identify research papers on A1 and A2 milk. Later he indicated that this was 'only producing a handful of papers but casein is producing a lot more.' On 19 June he sent NZFSA a draft of his report asking, 'Let me know how this is looking for what you are after.' Two days later Inkster forwarded some papers from Dairy Australia that they thought were relevant, and then on 17 July Swinburn sent his final draft ready to go out for peer review. Inkster responded: 'Terrific – thanks – we have no comments to add and would be pleased to see the report finalised.'

At the same time she advised that she had signed the copy of the contract, which in itself is perhaps surprising for a government contract, in that the job was already practically completed.

And then everything went quiet. Back in April 2003 Carole Inkster said on radio that she expected the report to be published by late May, but now the months were drifting by. In fact it was not until August 2004, 13 months after Boyd Swinburn supplied his draft, that the report was published.

Why did it take so long? Part of the answer is that it apparently took some time to get outside independent reviewers to approve the report for release. But a large part of the answer would seem to be that from NZFSA's point of view, the urgency had gone out of the matter. A2 Corporation had in the meantime been devastated by the deaths of Howard Paterson and Corran McLachlan, and was struggling to restructure. The new management had quickly realised that the court battles with Fonterra would drive them bankrupt and had withdrawn their claims. Basically, in terms of a threat to New Zealand's major export industry, the heat was off.

A few days before finally publicly releasing Boyd Swinburn's report, advance copies were sent to A2 Corporation, Fonterra and the New Zealand Commerce Commission. Then on 3 August 2004 the report was released. But an extremely important modification had been made in the intervening days. The NZFSA had decided to omit the Lay Summary at the front of the document. This Lay Summary summarised the major findings in two pages of non-technical language. Whereas the main report was written for scientists and policymakers, the Lay Summary was aimed at general citizens. Instead of focusing primarily on what government should do, it also focused on whether individual citizens should consider shifting to A2 milk.

Boyd Swinburn has confirmed to me that the Lay Summary was omitted without his approval or indeed without any discussion with him. In fact he did not know it had been omitted until I told him, the day after the report was released.

I had become aware of the omission through discussions with Andrew Clarke, the Chief Executive Officer of A2 Corporation. An A2 Corporation press release referred to statements by Boyd Swinburn that were not present in my publicly released copy. At my request, Andrew Clarke then sent me their pre-publication copy. What I then found was that not only had NZFSA omitted the Lay Summary, but it had subsequently repaginated the whole report, leaving extraordinarily large gaps between paragraphs in the technical Executive Summary, so that the overall length of the report (in pages) remained the same as when it contained the Lay Summary, and the main technical report started on the same page. It seemed to me to be a very clumsy attempt at covering up what it had done. But if I had not decided to pursue the matter the NZFSA would have got away with it, and the public would never have known that there had been such a report written to specifically address questions from its perspective.

When NZFSA released the report it put out its own press release stating its version of the major findings. It knew that most journalists would rely heavily on the press release rather than read though 43 pages of technical information.

Accordingly, the NZFSA said, 'There is no food safety issue with either type of milk' and this was widely reported in the media.' *Nowhere*, in fact, throughout the 43-page report did Professor Swinburn use the words 'safe' or 'safety' in relation to milk.

The press release also said, 'Professor Swinburn's review shows that there is insufficient evidence to demonstrate benefits of one type of milk protein over another'. Again, he never used those words either, nor indeed any words of equivalent meaning.

Then in a television interview Carole Inkster said, 'This report confirms our advice that it is very safe to drink any milk that's in the marketplace, A1 or A2.' Professor Swinburn made no statement like this either.

I was more than a little annoyed at the way the NZFSA was misrepresenting the information. Accordingly, I stated in radio and television interviews that I thought the NZFSA was putting a misleading spin on Professor Swinburn's findings. The 'misleading spin' claim was also widely reported in the print media.

I also asked NZFSA to release the Lay Summary. Although I already had a copy of it (obtained from A2 Corporation) this was strictly speaking a privileged document and I was uncomfortable about quoting it without getting official permission. I also wrote to Annette King, the Minister of Health, who had responsibility for NZFSA, indicating my displeasure and the reasons why.

My claims in the news media that the Lay Summary should be released were rejected by NZFSA. Carole Inkster said in a radio interview that there was no need to release the Lay Report, as everything was in the main report. But she did get herself into a bit of a tangle. She said, 'There is nothing that's being held back. The full text of the report is in the public arena. It's on our website.'

The presenter, Kevin Ikin, then asked, 'And that includes the Lay Summary, does it?'

Inkster replied, 'No, it doesn't include the Lay Summary because we felt it didn't add anything.'

Ikin then added, 'Carole Inkster says the Food Safety Authority does not intend to make the Lay Summary available.'

The NZFSA then got itself into an even bigger tangle when responding directly to me about my request for release of the Lay Summary under the Official Information Act. Carol Barnao, Director of Dairy and Plant Products at NZSFA, wrote to me that the Lay Report was 'not included in the final report, which is available on our website, as we feel that the tone is inconsistent with the substantive report.'

Now we are getting to the crux of the matter! Carole Inkster and Carol Barnao were contradicting each other as to the reasons for its non release. And how could NZFSA make judgement calls on what should and should not be released and then claim to be independent?

The tone of the Lay Summary was indeed somewhat different to the tone of the main report, and for a very good reason. In relation to public-health policy Boyd Swinburn was very clear that there was insufficient evidence to warrant warnings being placed on A1 milk. In the public health arena there is a need for an exceptionally high standard of proof before such a requirement can be made. But the risk-management issues are quite different at the level of individuals and the particular choices they make, and Boyd Swinburn's Lay Report, being aimed at ordinary citizens, reflected that.

So what did the Swinburn Report actually say? The final three paragraphs of the Lay Summary encapsulate the major message:

> The A1/A2 hypothesis is both intriguing and potentially very important for public health if it is proved correct. It should be taken seriously and further research is needed. In addition, the appropriate government agencies have a responsibility to communicate the current state of evidence to the public, including the uncertainty about the

> evidence. Further public health actions, such as changing dietary advice or requiring labelling of milk products, are not considered to be warranted at this stage. Monitoring is also required to ensure that any claims made for A2 milk fall within the regulations for food claims.
>
> Changing the dairy herds to more A2 producing cows is an option for the dairy and associated industries and these decisions will undoubtedly be made on a commercial basis. Changing dairy herds to more A2 producing cows may significantly improve public health, if the A1/A2 hypothesis is proved correct, and it is highly unlikely to do harm.
>
> As a matter of individual choice, people may wish to reduce or remove A1 beta-casein from their diet (or their children's diet) as a precautionary measure. This may be particularly relevant for those individuals who have or are at risk of the diseases mentioned (Type 1 diabetes, coronary heart disease, autism and schizophrenia). However, they should do so knowing that there is substantial uncertainty about the benefits of such an approach.

Eventually the NZFSA did relent, and following a parliamentary question from a member of the Green Party to Health Minister Annette King about this and related matters, it released the Lay Summary and put it on its website. From the NZFSA's perspective this was now the simplest thing to do, and it was a clever move, because it took the heat out of the issue. By this stage the report was old news and it was no longer going to make the front pages of the newspapers. (The Lay Summary is reprinted in this book as Appendix 3.)

So in many ways the NZFSA was successful. It had a report that had successfully communicated to most of the media that there was supposedly no problem with A1 milk (although in reality that was not what the report did say.) Important messages such as that the A1/A2 hypothesis is 'potentially very important for public health' were buried. The message that there was a need to communicate to the public the current state of evidence and the level of uncertainty, was also lost. And the call for publicly funded research was ignored.

It didn't take long before various dairy industry groups got on the bandwagon. Dairy Australia, the chief Australian industry organisation, had information on its website within 24 hours after the report was released, putting their particular spin on what Boyd Swinburn had allegedly said. And Kevin Wooding, Chair of Dairy Farmers of New Zealand said the report had 'settled the debate'. Really?

Professor Jim Mann from Otago University also weighed in to the debate, saying on National Radio that the report had produced nothing new. He said that any further research should be funded by commercial interests, not out of the public purse. This was a little puzzling, because Mann was at that time himself involved in publicly funded trials through Otago University funds, investigating the effect of A1 and A2 beta-casein on cholesterol. (This particular trial was discussed in Chapter 4.)

In the weeks immediately following the release of the report I was in regular contact with Boyd Swinburn. I had first talked to him a few months earlier, when I rang him in Australia to try and find out why his report was taking so long. From that discussion I was aware in broad terms of the tenor of his report and so there were no surprises. As soon as his report came out I emailed him again to confirm whether he had been involved in the decision to omit the Lay Summary, and also pointing out a number of relevant papers that he had not reviewed. By chance he was in Christchurch (where I live) running a course, and once he got that out of the way, and after several more email communications, we had two long meetings.

Several things emerged, both from the emails and the meetings. One was that, as previously indicated, he had *not* been party to any discussions about removing the Lay Summary. He said, 'I suspect they thought it was a bit more controversial and preferred to keep the debate dampened.' That particular interpretation I agree with 100%!

I felt there were several major omissions from his report and communicated my thoughts to him. My first email to him said:

> I felt you had missed some important work by Professor Cade and his group in relation to autism. Much of this may not have been picked up using the specific key words used by you, and may have required BCM or beta casomorphin or similar. I thought that inclusion of this work would have led to different conclusions in relation to autism and schizophrenia.
>
> I was also surprised that you didn't follow further down the track of the biochemistry and pharmacology of BCM, given that this is the peptide that distinguishes A1 and A2 milk. There is quite a lot of information on this, and it has been quite important in relation to my own judgements that there really is something important in the A2 hypothesis.

> I was also surprised that you didn't look at the small but potentially significant literature on LDL oxidation, and the importance of the tyr-pro-phe- sequence in that regard. This seems to go to the heart of the A2 hypothesis in relation to heart disease.

I was impressed by Swinburn's response, in that unlike so many of the people involved in the A1/A2 debate, he seemed genuinely open to new information, and to holding a rational debate aimed at increasing knowledge rather than supporting existing positions. As a consequence, we had two productive meetings from which I believe we both learned some things.

By this stage Swinburn was clearly frustrated with the way that NZFSA had released his report and the way that it had subsequently been misinterpreted by the media. Prior to its release, he had advised NZFSA that he would be in New Zealand and available to the media once the short course he was running was completed. However, NZFSA chose to go ahead and release the report anyway, without telling him, and at a time when he had said he would be unavailable. There was nothing that either he or I could do about this, but we did decide to write a joint email to Andrew Ferrier, the Chief Executive Officer (CEO) of Fonterra, to try and undo some of the damage.

Essentially, Boyd Swinburn's concern was that it seemed that the dairy industry was misinterpreting the risk-management issues. In particular, just because he was saying that at this stage ordinary milk containing A1 beta-casein did not need to carry a health warning, this did not mean that the A1/A2 issue should be ignored. So on 17 August 2004 I sent an email on behalf of both of us to Andrew Ferrier outlining those issues. It was headed *Risk Management Issues Relating to A2 milk* and included the following:

> Both Professor Swinburn and I believe that the report has been misinterpreted, and that the confusion has been compounded by the way in which NZFSA released the report without the Lay Summary. They then put their own interpretation on the findings that was actually quite different than what Professor Swinburn wrote. The Press Release by DCANZ (and other industry spokespeople) certainly seems to be based on misunderstandings.
>
> The focus of the Swinburn Report was to review evidence and provide advice in relation to public health. Professor Swinburn was quite clear that the level of proof was insufficient for any warning to

> be placed on milk, given that it is proper that regulators have to be very conservative in these matters.
>
> However, the risk management issues from a dairy industry perspective are quite different. If the industry thinks that the A1/A2 milk issue is essentially a non-issue then this would be quite incorrect. In this regard it is worth noting that Professor Swinburn focused on the evidence relating to humans and did not investigate a lot of the underlying science. Although this underlying science is highly relevant and provides major insights, using this type of evidence is not the way regulatory bodies work.
>
> We are aware that Fonterra has its own internal processes for assessing risk management, but we are also aware how internal groups within organisations can get locked into positions. We think this may be occurring, and would like the opportunity of presenting to you an outside perspective of where the evidence is actually leading ...

In response we received a letter, addressed to me but also copied by Fonterra to Boyd Swinburn, and written by Dr Joan Wright, General Counsel Regulatory Affairs at Fonterra. It included the following:

> Our Chief Executive officer, Andrew Ferrier, has asked me to respond to your email on the subject of Risk Management Issues relating to A1 and A2 milk dated 19 August 2004.
>
> Thank you for your interest and for raising your concerns. As you are aware the dairy industries in New Zealand and overseas have followed the scientific debate on the health effects of A1/A2 milk for a number of years.
>
> Fonterra previously commissioned a full review of the literature and research from an independent expert who advises that there is no convincing or probable evidence.
>
> - That A1 milk is a factor causing Type 1 diabetes or CHD; or
> - That A1 milk can cause autism or schizophrenia or its reduced consumption can improve autism or schizophrenia.
>
> Professor Swinburn's advice to NZFSA set out below, accords with the advice of national and international health experts and authorities:
>
> - Changes to dietary advice about milk consumption or food labelling of milk products are not warranted.
> - There is no need to change dairy herds to A2 producers.

There was no mention of the meeting that we sought. So there the matter rested. Boyd Swinburn and I had done our bit to try and ensure that incorrect messages were not becoming accepted as fact. But Fonterra was not really interested. I thought Fonterra's response, including some further comments to Boyd Swinburn and myself about sources of information and relevant expertise, was a little condescending, but perhaps that's normal for a big international company. In essence the reply confirmed that Fonterra had misinterpreted Boyd Swinburn's message. And it was apparent that it did not want to reconsider its position.

I subsequently wondered who Fonterra's 'independent expert' referred to by Joan Wright might have been. Initially I thought it was probably Professor Jim Mann. Certainly, when the media approached Fonterra for comment on health safety issues relating to A1 and A2 milk around this period they were directed to him. And sources within Fonterra have advised me that Jim Mann reviewed the A2 evidence back in the old NZ Dairy Board days, before Fonterra was formed.

Subsequently I wondered whether the expert was Jim Mann's colleague and co-author of a lot of his early work, Professor Stewart Truswell from Sydney University. Truswell was at that time the key external scientific witness being used by Fonterra in an unsuccessful attempt to overturn A2 Corporation's key genotyping patent (although at this stage the final ruling had not been made, and I had not been aware of any association between Truswell and Fonterra). Also, Truswell had in 2004 written (but not published until 2005) an article for the *European Journal of Clinical Nutrition* rubbishing the A2 hypothesis, although there was no disclosure in the published paper of any professional association with Fonterra. (Some of the Truswell arguments put forward in this article were discussed in Chapters 3 and 6, and others will come up in the final chapter.)

Given this situation I thought it would be interesting to find out the source of Fonterra's external advice. However, at the time I did not inquire further. I assumed from the tone of Joan Wright's letter, and the fact that she had chosen not to disclose the name, that they were keeping the identity 'in house'.

Eventually in March 2007 I did write back to Joan Wright seeking the identity of the 'independent expert'. But by then she had left Fonterra and the email bounced back. So I wrote directly to CEO Andrew Ferrier. He emailed back that I should talk to Jeremy Hill, to whom he copied his response. 'Jeremy is our Chief Technology Officer, and would be best to answer your inquiry. Regulatory affairs reports to Jeremy.'

Readers will recall that Hill features in many chapters of this book. And he subsequently confirmed that the independent witness was indeed Stewart Truswell. This in turn initiated some further correspondence, in which I reminded him that, at a meeting in August 2005, he had denied knowing of any association between Truswell and Fonterra. That further correspondence is also drawn upon in the next chapter.

A few months after the 2004 correspondence with Fonterra I had a brief discussion about A2 milk with Andrew Ferrier at a social event. My impression was that A2 milk was not an issue to which he had given a great deal of attention. This was not surprising, as he had only recently taken up the reins at Fonterra. In his previous job in Canada, which had nothing to do with the dairy industry, it would never have shown up on the radar. By the time of his arrival at Fonterra the issue had gone quiet, and chief executives of big international companies cannot be on top of every relevant issue. They have to rely on their organisation to keep them informed. Fonterra's problem would seem to be that senior managers may have relied too much on internal advice rather than exploring whether that advice and corporate stance needed independent review.

I have subsequently mentioned to three of the Fonterra directors, including the Chairman, that I think their company lacks the capacity to give sound unbiased advice on these matters to its senior executives and board of directors. I have said that I believe there are important risk-management issues that the directors need to be taking note of. They have not come back to me for further discussions. I have also made it very clear, when talking again to Andrew Ferrier in 2007, where I think the problem lies. But there are many things on his mind and I have not been able to get him to engage.

Some reflections

I believe that Boyd Swinburn undertook the inquiry with absolute integrity. Nevertheless, there were some major inadequacies. I believe he made a serious mistake at the start by thinking that he could do the work in only four days. It needed months, not days. In fact I think he probably did put in quite a lot more time than the allocated four days, but it was still nowhere near enough.

The way Boyd Swinburn went about the investigation was also far too limited. He missed a lot of the work by Professor Cade and his colleagues (outlined in Chapter 8). He also failed to investigate the underlying science. He found 38 relevant papers using the search words 'A1 milk', 'A2 milk' and 'casein', but failed to search for papers on the milk devil, BCM7. If he had done a search using the word 'casomorphin' he would have picked up over a hundred papers, many of them relevant. He also made no mention at all of issues surrounding milk intolerance. In the absence of all this material, inevitably the report was incomplete. There are at least 60 relevant papers and arguably a lot more that Boyd Swinburn did not consider. What would the outcome have been if all these papers had been considered?

The reason why Swinburn did not search out this information was because, as he and I said in our email to Andrew Ferrier, he 'focused on the evidence relating to humans and did not investigate a lot of the underlying science. Although this underlying science is highly relevant and provides major insights, using this type of evidence is not the way regulatory bodies work.'

Although this provides an accurate explanation, I do not regard it as a satisfactory justification. It was a tragedy for the advancement of knowledge that all the evidence was not considered.

The problem was then made much worse by the actions of the NZFSA in managing to bury the Lay Summary until it was 'stale news', and then by Fonterra's lack of interest in hearing what Swinburn had to say. And the way the NZFSA portrayed Swinburn's findings was totally unacceptable.

And so it is now time to move on and look at the business battles to get A2 milk to market within a very difficult regulatory environment. Hopefully some time in the future a food safety agency in some other country will decide to undertake a genuinely independent review. Perhaps a European country that has a high intake of A1 beta-casein (such as Finland), and also very high incidences of the diseases apparently associated with A1 beta-casein, will decide to do a review. Or perhaps a country like France, that has predominantly A2 dairy herds but is under major commercial pressure from countries producing A1 milk, will see both health and commercial advantages to be gained through reviewing these issues. Only time will tell.

NOTES

1 The inference is that this would be released to interested parties such as A2 Corporation and/or the media.

CHAPTER TWELVE

BUSINESS BATTLES: GETTING A2 MILK TO MARKET

Back in 2000 it must have seemed that it was all going to be so easy. The combination of the scientist Dr Corran McLachlan and the wealthy entrepreneur Howard Paterson seemed unstoppable. And behind them, as Chairman of the directors of the new company, there was the highly regarded Dunedin lawyer Jim Guthrie. Guthrie was a former Chair of the New Zealand Medical Council, the New Zealand Conservation Authority, and the New Zealand Law Society Resource Management Committee. What a combination of people! The market agreed and in no time the capitalisation of A2 Corporation on what was called the 'unlisted exchange' for start-up companies was NZ$61 million.[1] But as a stockbroker friend once advised me, biotechnology companies 'burn cash'. Getting new products to market is a huge challenge and the wayside is littered with failures. And when you are taking on the milk industry establishment, then it becomes a real David and Goliath battle – but with no guarantee that David will win.

In Chapter 1 I have already told much of the story leading up to the deaths of Corran McLachlan and Howard Paterson in 2003. With hindsight, there were plenty of problems in the months leading up to their deaths, but as long as Paterson was there with his money and his connections the overriding feeling was optimism.

It is hard to say exactly when the New Zealand Dairy Board decided to stand and fight on the issue of A2 milk but it was probably soon after the fateful meeting in October 2000 between Howard Paterson and NZ Dairy Board Chief Warren Larsen. It was at that meeting that phrases like 'class action' started to be thrown about by Howard Paterson in relation to non-disclosure of key information. Warren Larsen was clearly concerned that A2 Corporation was a bunch of irresponsible cowboys that could put the New Zealand dairy industry at risk. They needed to be stopped in their tracks.

Organisational culture can be very complex and power relationships can indeed be very subtle. But at some stage the word seemed to be spread throughout the NZ Dairy Board that A2 was a risk rather than an opportunity, and needed to be dealt with accordingly.

The years 2000 and 2001 were tumultuous times for the New Zealand dairy industry, with major restructuring. The old system, for the previous 70 years, had been based on lots of small co-operatives that processed raw milk into butter, cheese and other products which were then marketed by the NZ Dairy Board, a statutory marketing board that had both co-operative and government representatives. But the co-operatives had been rapidly amalgamating, until by 2000 there were only four of them left, two of which (the New Zealand Dairy Group and the Kiwi Dairy Co-operative) were processing about 95% of all dairy products. Both wanted to do their own marketing. Then in 2001 these two agreed to amalgamate, following what might be called an 'on-again-off-again' and then 'on-again' courtship. It was agreed among all parties, including the government, that the new mega co-operative would buy out the NZ Dairy Board shares owned by the other two minor co-operatives and each company (one large, the other two very small) would then do its own marketing. The government considered that statutory marketing boards had become outmoded, and was pleased to step back from any future involvement. Thus was formed the new mega co-operative, Fonterra.

Of course it wasn't all plain sailing, even after the merger details were thrashed out. There were lots of competing egos in the two amalgamating co-operatives and the NZ Dairy Board, and it took a while for the new structures to get bedded down. It is debatable how well-informed the leaders were about A2. They had their minds on other things. Almost certainly some misjudgements were made.

Prior to the 2001 industry restructuring, the NZ Dairy Board had also run the national breeding system, which included ranking the genetic merit of all the bulls used for artificial breeding. The Board had already decided to test the A1 and A2 status of all these bulls, so at least someone thought that A2 was a relevant issue.

However, the message farmers received from Fonterra was that A2 was something they should not worry about; indeed that A2 Corporation was irresponsible even to suggest that ordinary milk might have negative effects on health. As Lincoln University's professor of farm management and agribusiness, I decided – like most farmers – that A2 milk was something I did not need to bother about. History would show, I thought, that A2 Corporation was just a bunch of noisy entrepreneurs who were trying to stir up an unlikely story for their own advantage.

The first Annual Report from A2 Corporation was for the year ending 31 March 2001.[2] However, the accounts were not signed off until late August and the Chairman's Report was also probably written about then. The report reeked of optimism. Just a few months earlier, a share offer for six million shares at $2 each had been fully subscribed. The share prospectus had contained 'conservative' financial projections of burgeoning net surpluses before tax – reaching NZ$268 million by the year 2006! The alternative, higher estimate was for a surplus in 2006 of NZ$1.18 billion. This money was going to flow from DNA testing of cows and royalties on A2 milk products using A2 Corporation trademarks. The prospectus had pointed out that it was a speculative investment and that there were no guarantees. But the overall feeling was that things were going to happen.

In the 2001 Annual Report Chairman Jim Guthrie reported that: 'A2 Corporation is now separating out herds that produce pure A2 milk. Soon this milk and related products will be on supermarket shelves in New Zealand and Australia.' He also stated that the company had entered an exclusive license agreement with New Zealand Dairy Foods (a nationwide distributor and marketer) to put A2 milk on supermarket shelves by February 2002. (NZ Dairy Foods had been majority owned by the new Fonterra, but under a Commerce Commission ruling they were required to sell the company, and the divestment process was occurring during this period.)

Guthrie also laid out plans covering Australia, where 15,000 cows were being tested, and in Europe, where A2 Corporation Europe would be set up. He described forthcoming research programmes.

If there was a word of caution it was almost subliminal, and it related to the status of the patents. One of the key patents was for identifying A2 cows by testing their milk. This patent was originally owned jointly by the NZ Dairy Board and the Child Health Research Foundation, and arose directly from the work of Bob Elliott. A2 Corporation had bought a half-share in this patent from the Child Health Research Foundation. The other patent was for DNA testing of the cows using tail hairs, and was wholly owned by A2 Corporation. The problem was that the NZ Dairy Board was disputing this second patent, claiming that its own patent (now owned jointly with A2 Corporation) also covered this DNA testing. These issues were discussed in the memo from Jeremy Hill of 8 October 2000 (Chapter 1 and Appendix 2). Subsequent events proved Hill and the Dairy Board wrong, and the A2 Corporation patent was upheld in all the important jurisdictions, including the USA and Europe. In essence, the DNA patent owned by A2 Corporation has become the key patent, and the milk-testing patent has become much less important. But Fonterra, as successor to the NZ Dairy Board, continued to fight the patent battle through the courts for several years, and in relation to the Australian jurisdiction only withdrew in 2006.

Returning to the developing story from earlier in the decade, the 2002 Annual Report (signed off at the end of August 2002) was still upbeat. Chairman Jim Guthrie reported:

> You will have recently received my letter outlining the exciting results from the first of three major independent scientific investigations commissioned by A2 Corporation. This study, carried out by Professor Julie Campbell at the University of Queensland Centre for Research in Vascular Biology, has shown that consumption of A1 casein increases the risk of heart disease in rabbits whilst consumption of A2 casein does not. This is the strongest scientific evidence to date to support the epidemiological link between heart disease and consumption of A1 milk proteins.

One worry was that there was not yet any A2 milk on the supermarket shelves, either in New Zealand or Australia. CEO Corran McLachlan reported:

> The exclusive licence to sell A2 milk products in New Zealand which was granted to New Zealand Dairy Foods (NZDF) in 2001 has subsequently become non-exclusive due to their failure to bring A2 milk to market within the 14 month licence period. At the time the NZFDF licence was granted, A2 Corporation believed NZDF to be the ideal partner to promote and distribute A2 milk locally. Unfortunately a number of factors conspired to prevent NZDF bringing A2 milk to market within the required timeframe, the most significant being the extended sale process conducted by Fonterra for its majority stake in NZDF, and subsequently the Commerce Commission investigations into tendering of house brand milk supplies. Since the NZDF licence has become non-exclusive, A2 Corporation has subsequently executed

> non-exclusive local licences with several small to medium sized dairy producers, including an independent supermarket milk supplier and an organic yoghurt and cheese manufacturer.

One senses that Corran McLachlan might have liked to say more about the business forces at work that had led to NZDF deciding not to move forward with its licence. But of those matters we will never know. A few years later, in a complex business arrangement the NZDF brands were all repurchased by Fonterra.

The financial outcome for 2002 was that A2 Corporation had a financial deficit of NZ$2.9 million, in contrast to 'conservative projections' of a net operating surplus of $670,000. The company still had cash in hand but it was being used up very quickly.

The next episode began on 1 November 2002 with Deborah Hill Cone reporting in the *National Business Review*:

> Biotech company A2 Corporation has launched a High Court lawsuit against Fonterra Co-operative group accusing it of covering up the allegedly harmful effects of A1 milk, including research showing a link between 'bad milk' and mental disorders ... Documents obtained by the *National Business Review* show A2 will rely on a confidential Dairy Board (now Fonterra) memo from October 2000 in which top executives were warned by the group's own scientists there was growing evidence that peptides released from A1 milk may be related to the occurrence of some mental disorders ... [This is the Jeremy Hill memo reprinted as Appendix 2 of this book.]
>
> The lawsuit risks inflicting catastrophic damage to New Zealand's international reputation and foreign earnings as Fonterra turns over $14 billion and makes 20% of the country's total offshore receipts. As if that would not be enough of a PR disaster as the country tries to maintain its position as a clean, green food producer, A2 Corporation is going to ask the court under the Fair Trading Act to order Fonterra to put health warnings on its A1 milk setting out the risks of Type 1 diabetes, heart disease, autism and schizophrenia.
>
> A2 also wants the court to force Fonterra to publicly disclose all the information it has about the links between A1 milk and health risks.
>
> Barrister Julian Miles QC for A2 will argue Fonterra has been negligent in not warning the public about the research suggesting A1

> milk is unsafe for some people. A2 claims Fonterra has been materially influenced by its commercial objective of continuing to sell A1 milk and consumers of A1 milk are continuing to suffer from diseases of diabetes, heart disease, autism and schizophrenia as a result.

The response on national television that night from Fonterra spokesman and Research and Development Director Chris Mallett was that the information was 'well out of date ... A2's claims should not put people off normal milk. We think it is irresponsible because it neglects the very substantial health benefits it brings to people who consume it.' The television presenter then said, 'Fonterra says it will fight hard in court to protect its key product.'

One wonders how carefully A2 Corporation thought through its strategy. It probably made sense, but only as long as Howard Paterson was standing behind it with his financial muscle. Bringing biotechnology companies to market is not the only way to burn cash. Taking on a major company in legal proceedings isn't cheap.

The next media salvo was in the following week's *National Business Review*:

> Professor Garth Cooper, from the New Zealand Society for the Study of Diabetes, questioned some aspects of the most recent study, known as the Food and Diabetes Trial (FAD) which was published this year in the journal *Diabetologia*. The research has been used by Fonterra to undermine A2's research and back up its claim that there are no health risks with A1 milk. But Professor Cooper, who heads the human nutrition unit at the University of Auckland said he was surprised the FAD trial did not include any proof that the A1 and A2 caseins supplied by Fonterra were pure. In a crucially important trial of this nature, this was surprising as the entire research depended on the purity of the caseins. He would have expected detailed data to show these substances were scientifically pure: 'It worries me.'

This is indeed a fascinating report. If Professor Cooper had read the entire NZ Dairy Board memo of October 2000 he would have known that the Pregestimil had been found to contain BCM7. If he had then gone back and carefully read the FAD trial paper (discussed in Chapter 6), he would have realised that the trial was fatally confounded. Scientists do not usually slag each other in public, and so perhaps Cooper was politely telling the FAD scientists that they needed to admit they had a problem. But it is possible that he had not actually seen this memo in its entirety, because it had only been quoted selectively in the media. In that case his comments would be all the more perceptive and prescient.

Further in the same article, the *National Business Review* reported Fonterra's response to the previous week's article about the lawsuit. Craig Norgate, CEO of Fonterra at that time, was reported as saying, 'We would be the first to take a responsible public stand if we thought it was warranted'.

And then from Chris Mallett: 'There is no scientific evidence currently available to Fonterra, published or otherwise, which indicates A1 milk causes any of the negative health benefits claimed by A2 Corporation'.

I sometimes wonder whether that last statement may eventually come back to haunt Fonterra. To me, it does not seem consistent with the information provided in this book.

Then everything went quiet for a few weeks until the release in January 2003 of the Laugesen and Elliott paper in the *New Zealand Medical Journal*, (see Chapters 3 and 5) and the almost immediate response from the NZFSA that milk was 'still part of a balanced diet'.

A few weeks later attention shifted across to Australia, first with the launch by New South Wales dairy farmer and processor Phil Denniston, who was producing Fairbrae Jersey Gold A2 under license from A2 Corporation. This was the first time that A2 milk had been retailed anywhere in the world. Then at the end of March the Australian Broadcasting Corporation screened nationwide on Channel 2 the investigative documentary programme 'White Mischief' (see Chapter 1), which was introduced as follows:

> Milk ... as natural and wholesome as motherhood, packed with protein, vitamins and minerals, great for you and the kids. That's the image but just how beneficial is it. Now there are startling claims that the type of milk most Australians drink should carry a health warning. Filming in Australia, New Zealand and Britain's Channel Islands and drawing on data from more than a dozen countries, Four Corners tells a story of corporate intrigue, power games and cutting edge research.

'White Mischief' interviewed both the scientists and the entrepreneurs. Some scientists such as Professor Sir John Scott were highly supportive; others such as Professor Len Harrison were sceptical. There were shots of Howard Paterson flying around his farms by helicopter and of Corran McLachlan inspecting some of his rare book collection, and talking of the Goldie painting he had sold to generate funds. It made great viewing but drew no conclusions.

The final sound bite from Howard Paterson was about questions of evidence and proof: 'If you actually line all the evidence up, you've got a situation there where, you know, it's got a tail, it's got four legs, big white teeth, it barks and answers to Rover. You know, it's pretty obvious to me that it's a dog.'

And then there was a sound bite from former NZ Dairy Board Chief Warren Larsen: 'They've [A2 Corporation] travelled a path which has caused a lot of concern in the public. The public, then, are left in a position where they have to make a judgement on who to trust. And I leave you to make that call.'

Regardless of how one judged the evidence, there was no doubt that A2 Corporation was getting lots of publicity.

A few weeks later A2 milk became available in New Zealand, first produced by Klondyke Dairies in Christchurch and Ridge Natural Foods Ltd in Hamilton. Subsequently, Fresha Valley became a second North Island franchisee. But Fonterra was not sitting back. It purchased some A2 milk processed by Klondyke Dairies which was labelled 'Just A2', had it tested in Australia, and claimed that it contained some A1. It has subsequently been shown that the particular technique used (a CE test) is actually unreliable in regard to low-level contamination and regularly gives false positives, i.e. shows a small percentage of A1 when there is actually none. I have seen later test results from Food Science Australia confirming this: the test gives false results that milk from pure A2 individual cows is only about 90% A2. As explained in Chapter 10, this is impossible: individuals can only be 0%, 50% or 100%. But A2 Corporation and Klondyke Dairies could not guarantee at the time that the milk was totally free of A1 milk, i.e. that there was no chance of there being a single A1 cow in the A2 herds. Indeed Dr Andrew Clarke from A2 Corporation says that at the time they were not even given the opportunity of presenting counter-evidence. Instead the Commerce Commission required them to change the labelling. And there was further negative publicity for A2 Corporation with the NZFSA advising that all milk was safe. Over in Australia, Dr Peter Clifton from the Nutrition Clinic of CSIRO was reported in the news media as saying,

'There's absolutely no evidence that milk is related to diabetes, autism, or any of these conditions.'

Really? Then what is all the material presented in this book? There may be debate as to whether or not there is proof, but to suggest there is 'no evidence' would seem amazing. However, this is the message that Australian citizens received.[3]

It was a crucial time for A2 Corporation and their franchisees, with a need to increase the scale of operations to ensure long-term viability. Low volumes mean high unit costs, which mean high prices. And high prices work against high volumes. There is only one way to break out of that cycle and it is to promote. The problem for the franchisees was that they did not have the resources to do the promotion. In any case, borrowing to fund their own promotion of A2 milk would have been a dangerous strategy, given that their franchises were non-exclusive. And A2 Corporation itself was still burning cash through funding of research, developing an international strategy and paying big fees to its patent lawyers. Getting the promotion message right was always going to be tough because consumer laws in both Australia and New Zealand prevented marketers from making negative health claims in relation to A1 milk. It was a tricky business.

Howard Paterson and Corran McLachlan knew they needed to get more capital and had plans to raise it. One of the franchisees has told me that Paterson said not to worry: that he meant to support this business to ensure that it broke through any development problems. And when Howard Paterson said something like that he meant it. No Paterson business had ever failed.

Then everything went wrong. First it was Howard Paterson who died by choking on a chip in his Fiji hotel room. It sounds such an unlikely story, but as I explained in Chapter 1, it happens to be true. And then Corran McLachlan succumbed to secondary tumours from a melanoma. What a disaster! Chairman Jim Guthrie was left to pick up the pieces, to get a new chief executive officer and to find some more directors. Perhaps most importantly of all, with Howard Paterson no longer there, the funding stream was suddenly gone.

The 2003 Annual Report of A2 Corporation makes grim reading. It contains eulogies to Howard Paterson and Corran McLachlan. It also introduces Andrew Clarke, previously a scientist with the company, as the new CEO. It reported a financial deficit for the year to 31 March of NZ$2.16 million, with current assets exceeding current liabilities by only

$139,000. The report was signed off in November. Reading between the lines the company must by that time have been insolvent were it not for the directors' guarantees. A capital-raising exercise was planned.

There was some good news in late 2003. In November A2 Corporation announced it had linked with IdeaSphere in the USA. According to website reports, this would 'see A2 milk sold in over 5000 US retail health food outlets'. Jim Guthrie was quoted as saying that the agreement would result in 'minimum royalty payments in the first year of $1 million and $4 million in the second year.' News reports also quoted Guthrie as saying if A2 did not make it in the USA with this partnership in a market used to buying health and nutritional products, it would not make it anywhere.

So what is IdeaSphere? According to an article in *Natural Foods Merchandiser* in 2004 by Jim Aguilar, 'You won't find much about IdeaSphere in the press. And forget about checking its website – it doesn't have one.' But apparently it does have excellent access to finance. According to Aguilar, its principal owners included (and presumably still do include) Amway heir Dave Van Andel; celebrity motivational speaker Anthony Robbins; Peter Lusk, who is vice chairman of a US$1.5 billion hedge fund; and Mark Fox, who is the President of IdeaSphere itself.

IdeaSphere is a key player in the health and wellness industry. Fox estimated in early 2004 that IdeaSphere company revenues could exceed US$200 million that year. Key assets and brands of IdeaSphere include Twinlab, Nature's Herbs, Alvita Taes brands and Rebus Publishing.

Then, in Australia, A2 Corporation licensed an independent start-up company called A2 Dairy Marketers Pty Ltd to market A2 milk Australia-wide.

A2 Corporation accounts for the 12 months ending 31 March 2004 showed a negative net cash flow from operating activities of NZ$1.47 million. The consolidated loss after amortisation of patents was NZ$2.16 million. Cash inflows included a $625,000 bank loan and there was an overdraft of $602,000. So the company was still burning through the cash, with minimal revenue coming in.

In April 2004 A2 Corporation undertook a renounceable share offer of two additional A2 shares at 5 cents each. Existing shareholders could either purchase these shares themselves for 5 cents or sell the purchase rights to other people. This raised about NZ$2.9 million. The offer documents for the renounceable-rights issue stated that the business model was to license the company's intellectual property to the most suitable partners in various parts of the world. The company would derive its revenues from testing cows and from royalties on the sale of A2 milk. The documents stated that although New Zealand was important for several reasons (which were not actually stated), from a revenue perspective it would not be significant when compared to potential markets elsewhere. Australia, North America, Europe and Asia were all identified and discussed as important markets. No dividends were expected to be paid to shareholders for at least 24 months.

In May 2004 there was a considerable restructuring of major shareholdings. Corran McLachlan had held his shares through a private company, Machin Investments, which was principally owned by himself and Peter Hinton. The ownership of Machin Investments changed, with Cliff Cook, in partnership with Greg Hinton, buying a majority of these shares. Cliff Cook had been in the healthcare industry since 1976 and was a major shareholder and Deputy Chair of Metlifecare, which owned retirement villages and rest homes. Both Cliff Cook and Greg Hinton joined the Board of Directors of A2 Corporation. Cliff then became Chair of A2 Corporation when Jim Guthrie stood down. Guthrie had been suffering from Parkinson's disease for 12 years and said it was now time for him to step back from the front line. In fact Cliff Cook had already been playing a key behind-the-scenes role, in that the major bank loan and overdraft were guaranteed by his private family companies. A2 Corporation was so weak financially that the only way it could get the loans was by Cliff Cook agreeing to act as guarantor to the bank if A2 Corporation went into liquidation.

The 2004 calendar year continued to be tumultuous. In August the NZFSA Report brought A2 milk back into the news (see Chapter 11). Then, just as that little furore died down, Australian franchisee A2 Dairy Marketers hit the headlines. First it was via a 'Matters of Public Interest' speech by Mr Hopper, the member for Darling Downs in the Queensland Legislative Assembly (the state parliament). It was a rip-roaring endorsement of A2 Dairy Marketers. He described how the mainstream dairy industry had been doing

> ... everything in its power to ensure A2 milk's launch into the market place was an extremely difficult one, with complaints being made by the industry bodies and subsequent investigations by Queensland Health and the ACCC. Major dairy companies are also going to great lengths to say that farmers who dual supply A2 milk will not have their milk collected on farm.

He called A2 Dairy Marketers 'a great company', and said that the NZFSA had 'misled the public of New Zealand into believing that [Professor] Swinburn had concluded that A1 milk was safe.' And he concluded, 'I say that the big companies are running scared.'

A few weeks later, on 9 September 2004 De-Anne Kelly, who was a member of the Australian Federal Parliament and also the Parliamentary Secretary for the Minister of Transport and Regional Services, announced federal funding of AU$1.3 million to be provided to A2 Dairy Marketers to help it to establish a processing facility on the Atherton Tablelands, inland from Cairns. This was an area where dairy farmers were struggling financially and the prospect of receiving a premium for A2 milk was very attractive. It wasn't too far out from the next Australian election and in good old 'pork barrelling' political style it was time for some largesse. It seemed that A2 Dairy Marketers were in the right place at the right time.

Some sections of the Australian news media were a little cynical, and also wondered whether De-Anne Kelly was in danger of making a fool of herself. They asked whether she knew that A2 Dairy Marketers were about to come up in court on a charge of misleading advertising. De-Anne Kelly confirmed that she knew this was about to happen, but said it was important to get on and do something. Also, she said she had the support of both sides of the Queensland state parliament.

Sure enough, a few weeks later, A2 Dairy Marketers came up in the Brisbane Court. On 30 September 2004 the Brisbane daily newspaper, *The Courier Mail*, reported, 'Queensland Health argued that the company's claim that A2 milk was more beneficial to health than regular milk was likely to mislead consumers. The company was fined $15,000.'

Technically A2 Dairy Marketers was guilty, and indeed it pleaded guilty. It had stepped over the line in its advertising, and instead of simply saying how good its product was, it had indicated there was a problem with mainstream milk. We may supposedly live in a world of free speech, but making negative claims in advertising that someone else's product has something wrong with it is not allowed. And that applies even if the message is correct. However, I was surprised that A2 Dairy Marketers did not fight the case, because its guilt seemed to be technical rather than moral, and it had plenty of evidence for what it had said. But of course it would have cost a great deal of money. Small start-up companies have to be very careful in choosing which battles to fight when the opponent has very deep pockets.

I decided to ring the managing director, Lindsay Stewart, to try to find out more about what was happening. The conversation surprised me greatly. Lindsay told me that he needed half a million dollars within 48 hours if his business was to survive. Now hold on a minute, I responded, I thought you had been fined $15,000. Yes, was the reply, but we need half a million dollars immediately. In fact it became apparent over the next few days that they needed more than a million dollars. It seems that it was a classic case of some entrepreneurs who had got out of their business depth. A2 Dairy Marketers had run out of money, and that had very little to do with the court case – although it may well have been the reason it decided not to fight the court case. A few days later A2 Dairy Marketers went into receivership.

Here was another crisis for A2 Corporation back in New Zealand. A2 Corporation had no ownership of A2 Dairy Marketers, which was simply the main Australian franchise holder, licensed to use the A2 trademarks for a fee on each litre of milk sold. A2 Dairy Marketers had made good progress in the Brisbane market and was about to move into other states as well as Queensland. The licence fees were A2 Corporation's major source of income at this stage. It would be a strategic disaster if the marketing of A2 were to fall over. So A2 Corporation quickly stepped in, rolled up its sleeves, and within a few weeks had A2 milk back in the supermarkets throughout southern Queensland. But this time A2 Corporation was in control and A2 Dairy Marketers Pty Ltd no longer existed.

Getting directly involved in marketing milk had not been part of the business plan of A2 Corporation. Despite the recent capital raising, money was still very tight. So A2 Corporation saw its involvement only as a short-term strategy until it could attract a much larger investor. This did not take long, and in January 2005 A2 Corporation announced an agreement to sell the new Australian subsidiary company A2 Australia Pty Ltd to the large Singapore-based food and beverage company Fraser & Neave. This was an exciting step. Fraser & Neave had assets of about SG$8 billion, operated in about 20 countries and had 11,000 employees. Clearly it was big enough to make such an operation work.

The year 2005 under Fraser & Neave's management was one of quiet progress in the Australian market. This must have been a great relief after the shambles of 2004. By the end of the year the milk was available in more than 600 supermarkets and convenience stores throughout all states of mainland Australia. Weekly sales rose to about 100,000 litres.

But despite the wide availability there was not a great deal of promotion. By the end of 2005 my Australian friends were telling me it was not difficult to find A2 milk in the shops, but unless you were looking for it you would probably never realise it was there. Selling 100,000 litres a week may sound impressive but it is well under 1% of the fresh milk market.

The problem of how to promote A2 milk is encapsulated in comments by Phil Denniston of Fairbrae Milk. It will be recalled that Fairbrae Milk was Australia's original A2 franchisee. Throughout 2005 Fairbrae was still battling away, selling A2 milk along the eastern seaboard from its base in the Northern Rivers region of New South Wales. Denniston wrote as follows on the Fairbrae website:

> **A2 Milk -- the debate (or lack there of by restricting debate)**
> In a recent report to the New Zealand Food Authority on Beta-casein A1 and A2 in milk, Professor Boyd Swinburn, Professor of Public Health Nutrition at the School of Health Sciences, Deakin University, Melbourne, makes it clear that A2 Milk cannot be ignored.
>
> ... Unfortunately we cannot provide you with access to this report by link because NSW Safe Food has indicated it would prosecute us. NSW Safe Food is arguing that our home page constitutes an 'Advertisement' under the Act and that if we provide any link to another home page that gives scientific information on the debate about A2 Milk, then that link is part of our 'Advertisement'.
>
> The Act basically prohibits the mentioning of any disease or medical condition or words like 'Health' in any advertisement or on any food label. Thus if a link we provide mentions any disease or condition of human health that is being linked to consumption of normal milk, it is currently being treated as part of our 'advertisement'.
>
> We do not agree - but can't risk a fine of up to $250,000. We also know that there are food producers and promoters who are blatantly ignoring this regulation. Why have we been singled out one might ask? We don't mind being required to comply with the law provided everyone else has the same rules applied. No doubt it is because of the financial and political power of the established milk producer in Australia! The Dairy Industry is obviously very nervous about A2 milk. The pressure being applied by it on us is presently by complaint to the NSW Safe Food Authority.
>
> Do a search on the net for 'A2 milk' – you will find a wealth of

> technical debate and references – make your own mind up! According to our customer feed back A2 milk does make a difference for a lot of people with a variety of conditions – and that's about all we are permitted to say without risking prosecution.

A2 Corporation was wrestling with similar issues itself in relation to its website material. CEO Andrew Clarke had to weave a very careful path to avoid the ire of the New Zealand Commerce Commission.

In the meantime, progress by and with IdeaSphere in developing American markets had been slow. The IdeaSphere agreement required payments to be made to A2 Corporation during the time that A2 milk was being brought to market in the USA. In early 2005 it became clear that IdeaSphere had reneged on a payment of US$400,000. Things did not look good. However, the agreement was renegotiated on the basis that A2 Corporation would become partner in a Delaware-registered company called A2 Milk Company LLC and they would develop the market together. This too represented a fundamental change of business policy, and needed more capital.

Existing shareholders were by now very reluctant to keep supplying more capital, and the 2005 renounceable-rights issue was undersubscribed. This had been foreseen, and Cliff Cook and business interests linked to him stepped up by underwriting the capital issue. It meant that Cook and his business interests now owned 51% of A2 Corporation through the company Mountain Road Investments Ltd, which he controlled.

A lot of planning had to go into devising a marketing strategy for the American market. But eventually, in April 2007, A2 milk was launched in seven midwestern states of the USA by The Original Foods Company through the Hy-Vee supermarket chain. Hy-Vee has some 200 supermarkets in Nebraska, Iowa, Kansas, Illinois, Missouri, South Dakota and Minnesota.

The positioning strategy for A2 milk in the USA is to market it as a natural premium-quality milk. Accordingly, it is produced only from cows that have not been treated with the synthetic hormone recombinant bovine somatotropin (rbST).

It may come as a surprise to non-Americans, and even indeed to most American consumers, that mainstream American milk comes predominantly from cows that are fed a special growth hormone. rbST causes cows to produce more milk, but it also increases infection in their udders (mastitis) and reduces fertility. However, there are no proven effects on humans from drinking the milk from rbST-treated cows. In New Zealand, Australia and Europe it is banned, but the Americans see it differently.

One of the ironies of food marketing is that, given that A2 milk in the USA is being advertised as coming only from cows that have not been treated with rbST, American labelling law requires them to add the statement that the 'FDA states no significant difference has been shown between milk derived from rbST treated and non-rbST treated cows.' However, there is no requirement for competitors to mention that their milk is from rbST-treated cows, and that this increases udder infections and lowers cow fertility![4]

There will be other challenges in marketing A2 milk in the USA. For example, as in Australia and New Zealand, A2 promoters have to be very careful about suggesting their competitors' milk might be associated with health problems. Accordingly, the American advertising makes no mention of any of the health conditions described in this book.

In the meantime there were further developments in Australia, with A2 Corporation buying back in April 2006 the company A2 Australia Pty Ltd from Fraser & Neave. It appears that A2 Corporation became impatient with the rate at which Fraser & Neave were developing the market and so decided to get more closely involved itself. Then, in December 2006, A2 Corporation announced it was in negotiations with So Natural Foods Australia Limited for a joint venture to develop both the Australian and Japanese markets. 'So Natural Foods', subsequently rebadged as 'Freedom Nutritional Products' (FNP), is listed on the Australian Stock Exchange. It has a range of supermarket products including soy milk and canned seafoods. It also specialises in health-focused nutritional products sold through gyms and sports centres. Its Australian brands include 'Freedom' and 'So Natural'. It also has the 'Thorpedo' brand of food and nutritional products sold in Japan. A 50/50 joint venture between FNP and A2 Corporation was confirmed in May 2007.

The key driver of recent developments at A2 Corporation has been Chairman of the Board and major shareholder Cliff Cook. Cook has the financial resources to make things happen. In that regard it is somewhat like the old days with Howard Paterson. However, the one remaining difference – and it is a big one – is that at this stage the broader market is not following Cook in the way it followed wherever Howard Paterson went. This means that Cook has himself become very much the dominant shareholder in the company. But without him the company would almost certainly no longer exist.

In among all these activities the marketing situation within New Zealand itself remained subdued. There had been tension between A2 Corporation and at least one of the two remaining franchisees (Ridge and Fresha Valley) in relation to promotion and who should be doing it. It had become clear that the business model they were using was fundamentally flawed. The franchisees were prepared to promote their own products but it made little sense for them to promote the generic issue of A2 milk when their franchises were non-exclusive. And A2 Corporation itself lacked the necessary capital. By early 2007 A2 Corporation and its franchisees had retreated, at least temporarily, to the north of the North Island plus just one outlet in Wellington and one in Dunedin.

Looking back, it is easy to see why A2 Corporation has struggled. It truly has been a David and Goliath battle. It is also clear that A2 Corporation, at least for three critical years from 2003 through to 2006, was seriously hampered by lack of capital. If there is one message I will be giving to my agribusiness students back at Lincoln University, it is about the cost of carving out a market niche, particularly when the existing players see you as a threat.

Marketing of A2 milk is very much a story on the move. At the A2 Corporation Annual General Meeting in July 2006 it was reported that A2 milk was available in Australia in more than a thousand stores, including 800 supermarkets. This was 400 more than was being reported just a few months earlier. However, it was not clear whether milk sales were actually increasing. And then, in February 2007 A2 Corporation announced it had appointed a new CEO, Anthony Lawler, a former mid-level Fonterra executive. A2 Corporation advised that the new appointment was consistent with a transformation from a biotech start-up company to an FMCG (fast-moving consumer goods) company.

In June 2007 A2 Corporation released its interim report for the 2007 financial year. It reported increased income of NZ$7.6 million which was more than a fivefold increase over the previous year. But it also reported a more than fourfold increase in the net loss of over NZ$5 million. However, the accompanying report, titled 'A2 set to capitalise on strong global sales platform' captured the attention of the market. In just a few days the capitalised value of the company more than doubled to almost NZ$60 million. Shares rose to over 40 cents. It was only a few months earlier they had sold as low as 6 cents!

Fonterra itself has had very little to say in public in recent years. This appears to be a deliberate strategy. However, behind the scenes it has continued its efforts to influence key people. For example I have a 12-page briefing paper on Fonterra letterhead sent by the company to an American journalist in late 2004 or early 2005. (The document itself is dated September 2003 but the computer file also carries the edit history, with the last edit being from Research and Development Director Chris Mallett's computer on 15 June 2004.) It says, 'Fonterra believes that A2 Corporation's claims are irresponsible because they may result in normal people removing milk from their diet to the detriment of their overall health and well-being.' It also says that:

> There is no valid scientific evidence, currently available to Fonterra, published or otherwise, that milk with the A1 beta-casein causes the negative health effects claimed by A2 Corporation ... Fonterra has conducted itself in a transparent and open manner when dealing with this issue ... Fonterra completely rejects any claims by A2 Corporation that it has been secretive.

It seems that Fonterra is unlikely to change its position in the near future. In March 2007 I engaged in several rounds of email correspondence with Jeremy Hill, who had responsibility for regulatory affairs within Fonterra. His final statement was:

> I remain convinced that this is not something that Fonterra can afford to devote significant attention to.
>
> When A2 Corporation or any one else can convince the mainstream health or medical bodies that the issue is a concern, or scientific evidence is produced that convinces me to change my position, then I will recommend that Fonterra does indeed take this area seriously.

From other sources in Fonterra my understanding is that it is indeed keeping a watching brief on A2, and that it does have a plan to put into action if necessary. I hope it does not include shooting the messenger. What I do know is that Fonterra still sees A2 as a risk rather than an opportunity. And to me, that seems a huge pity.

It is also important to understand that the only key assets that A2 Corporation has are its intellectual property. It has exclusive patents for testing animals, plus a range of trademarks covering the branding of A2 milk. It therefore has the exclusive right in many countries to market milk labelled as 'A2 milk'. But it cannot stop other big players from selling milk produced from herds that are exclusively A2 cows, and labelling this milk as 'free from A1 beta-casein'. This is because A2 Corporation does not and cannot own the A2 variant of the gene. It is a natural gene.

One of the ironies is that the business side of the story could so easily have been different. Just two weeks before Howard Paterson's death in 2003, Fonterra had reached a handshake agreement with him as to how they could stop fighting in the courts and work together to develop A2 milk. Remember that Paterson was, among many other things, New Zealand's and possibly the world's largest dairy farmer. As well as being the A2 Corporation financier he was also Fonterra's largest shareholder and milk supplier. Paterson could stitch up deals that no-one else could. And this was a very special deal that relied on the trust that was in Paterson's handshake. With him no longer there, Fonterra walked away.

So what will the future bring? Crystal-ball gazing is always a risky pursuit. Whether A2 Corporation can break through and become a profitable company remains uncertain. Clearly a lot will depend on what happens in the USA and Australia. A2 Corporation is going to need more partners if it is to take on the world. Will Fonterra be one of them? If the ball really starts rolling then it will not stop. Perhaps it has already started.

NOTES

1 This is the figure obtained if the market price per share is multiplied by the total number of shares to give a total value of the company.

2 It is normal practice for New Zealand companies to operate on a 1 April to 31 March financial year. This means, for example, that the 2001 financial year includes nine calendar months of 2000 and three calendar months of 2001.

3 Dr Peter Clifton is also an author of CSIRO's extremely popular but controversial book The CSIRO *Total Wellbeing Diet*. *Nature*, which many consider the world's pre-eminent science journal, was moved to write an editorial in December 2005 where they described the marketing claims that this diet is 'scientifically proven' as being 'decidedly unsavoury'.

4 It is widely accepted amongst veterinarians and agriculturalists that the very high cow replacement rates on American dairy farms are associated with the use of rbST, which reduces the productive lives of the cows because of more udder infections, reduced fertility and increased lameness. But the practice of injecting rbST continues because of the increased milk production, and in essence is economically driven.

CHAPTER THIRTEEN

BRINGING IT ALL TOGETHER

I have now presented all of the evidence I am aware of both for and against the A2 hypothesis. In this final chapter I will bring together and summarise that evidence. Then it is up to readers to draw their own conclusions.

But first there is one more issue to briefly explore. It is the importance or otherwise of milk to a balanced diet. I have given considerable thought as to whether this is an issue I want to get involved in. However, it is clearly an issue that has influenced the New Zealand Food Safety Authority in its response to concerns about A1 beta-casein. In essence, the argument is that we must not do anything that would lead people to drink less milk, because milk is so important to a balanced diet. Of course the proponents of A2 milk have never said that people should stop drinking milk. They have just said that people should drink A2 milk, not A1. But I do want to clarify a few things about milk consumption.

It is only in the last two thousand years that humans have drunk large quantities of cows' milk. It was certainly not part of the traditional hunter/gatherer diet. Today in many parts of the world cows' milk is still only a very minor part of the diet. Also, in many of these low-milk countries, diseases that are often associated with a lack of calcium (e.g. osteoporosis) are uncommon. So although milk is a very important and valuable source of nutrients, particularly for children, it is difficult to argue that it is *essential for adults*. It is definitely a valuable source of many nutrients, but there are alternatives. If you want to look at the milk debate more closely, see the website of the Harvard School of Public Health at Harvard University (www.hsph.harvard.edu). You may be surprised to see what is written there.

So now it is time to review the A2 evidence. The starting point is the remarkable epidemiological evidence. The peer-reviewed scientific evidence is clear: there is a remarkably strong association between countries that have high intakes of A1 beta-casein and the incidence of Type 1 diabetes and heart disease. These associations are statistically extremely strong, so we know with a very high level of certainty that they are not due to random factors. As to what could be causing such an association, no credible alternative explanations have been put forward. Efforts to find alternative factors that could be causative have been likewise unsuccessful. Using the fundamental scientific concept of accepting the simplest scientific theory that fits the data, then the best theory would seem to be that A1 beta-casein is an important factor in both Type 1 diabetes and heart disease.

The second piece of evidence is centred around the fact that A1 beta-casein and A2 beta-casein are digested differently, despite having only one different amino acid out of 209. The evidence for this is both theoretical (relating to the strength of the bonds which proline forms with other amino acids) and from empirical research by at least three laboratories. This evidence shows that in the test tube when digestive enzymes are added to A1 beta-casein there is a large release of BCM7, whereas this does not happen with A2 beta-casein.

The third piece of evidence is that BCM7 is known for a fact to be a powerful opioid. This has been known for many years from laboratory work. The effects have also been clearly demonstrated when BCM7 is injected into rats. It has further been shown that the effects can be countered by the administration of naloxone, an opioid antagonist.

The fourth piece of evidence is that the incidence of Type 1 diabetes in naturally susceptible genotypes of mice and rats is higher when they are fed A1 beta-casein than when they are fed A2 beta-casein. The strength of this relationship is stronger in some trials than others, but in all published trials to date, including the Food and Diabetes (FAD) trial (which included undisclosed diet confounding), there was positive evidence of this association.

The fifth piece of evidence is that rabbits fed A1 beta-casein develop considerably more arterial plaque on their aorta than do similarly treated rabbits fed A2 beta-casein. This happens over a period of just a few weeks.

The sixth piece of evidence comprises a broad range of data from American and European investigations showing that autistic and schizophrenic persons typically excrete large quantities of BCM7 in their urine. The only known source of this peptide is casein. When these people are placed on a milk-free diet the excretion of the peptide declines markedly and there is an easing of their symptoms. There is a strong presumption that the reason these people are particularly susceptible to BCM7 is that they have an impaired digestive system, enabling the peptide to cross the intestinal wall and enter the blood.

The seventh piece of evidence relates to explanations of the mechanisms that might be causing these diseases. In the case of Type 1 diabetes, an auto-immune disease in which the body destroys its own insulin-producing cells, it seems that the body gets confused between BCM7 and a very similar molecule in the insulin-producing cells. In the case of heart disease, the mechanism appears to be related to the oxidant properties of BCM7, although that may be only part of the story. And in relation to autism and schizophrenia, the apparent explanation relates to the known opioid effects of BCM7. It is highly likely that not only does the BCM7 cause immediate behavioural effects but that it also affects the way the brain develops.

The reason why only some people are affected by BCM7 is likely to relate to whether they either currently have, or previously had at some crucial time of their lives, an impaired digestive system allowing BCM7 to enter the bloodstream. The very strong evidence that people with stomach ulcers have unusually high levels of heart disease when placed on a high-milk diet further corroborates this. Similarly, the evidence that sufferers of untreated coeliac disease, Crohn's disease and ulcerative colitis can have high levels of mental disorders is consistent with such an explanation.

Another piece of evidence relates to the differences in the antibodies to casein, A1 beta-casein and A2 beta-casein amongst sufferers of various diseases compared to people without these diseases.

Finally, there is the anecdotal evidence of people who have moved to milk that is free of A1 beta-casein. Are they all wrong?

The counter-evidence seems remarkably scanty. It seems that elevated cholesterol levels are unlikely to be a prime link in the chain of events by which the milk devil does its nasty work. There are two short-term human trials which have found no evidence of such a link. But then, there was never any obvious reason why cholesterol would be the mechanism. The trials with rabbits did show a cholesterol effect but this could have been a secondary outcome. When everything else is going wrong in the body, then this can have an impact on cholesterol levels.

Where else is the counter-evidence? I cannot find anything credible in the scientific literature.

However, although I cannot find anything else that is credible, at least some sections of the establishment are still mounting arguments against A2. Therefore it is only fair that I present these arguments, even if they do appear, at least to me, to lack credibility.

The scientist who has recently come to the fore in making these arguments is Professor Stewart Truswell, who has already been mentioned in Chapters 3, 6 and 11 of this book. He has been publishing in the medical literature since 1957 on a broad range of topics. Fonterra described him as 'the senior professor of human nutrition in Australia' when putting him forward as their expert witness in an unsuccessful attempt to overturn the A2 Corporation genotyping patent in 2004/05. Professor Truswell has expressed his views to the scientific community in a paper published in 2005 in the *European Journal of Clinical Nutrition* (*EJCN*). Subsequently in 2006 the *EJCN* published a response from me, and also a joint one from Dr Andrew Clarke (A2 Corporation's Chief Executive Officer at that time) and Dr Jock Allison (an A2 Corporation director). And subsequently to that Truswell responded with his author's right of reply.[1]

So what did Truswell say? First he described the hypothesis linking A1 beta-casein to a range of diseases as 'ingenious', then he tore it apart. He started with the epidemiology relating to Type 1 diabetes. Essentially, his argument was that these sorts of studies never prove anything by themselves, and should not be taken as proof without supporting evidence. On that point there can be no disagreement. The epidemiology provides very strong evidence but not absolute proof.

Truswell then went on to present the FAD trial with rats and mice that was discussed in detail in Chapter 6. He talked about the 'meticulous' methodology and the 'distinguished international panel of authors'. He failed to mention the non-disclosure of diet confounding. (At the time of his 2005 paper it is possible that he was unaware of this confounding, but in his 2006 response to my published letter, in which this issue was pointed out, he still chose to ignore it.) He stated that with the Biobreeding BB rats 'there was little difference between A1 and A2 beta-caseins and that none were significant.' This is wrong. The non-confounded diets using the Prosobee base did show a statistically significant higher level of diabetes in rats fed A1 beta-casein compared to rats fed A2 beta-casein (46% versus 19%). In his 2006 response he says that 'any reader of the literature must surely take the findings of experienced researchers in Ottawa, London (England) and Auckland as the latest (perhaps the final) word on the subject.' He also repeats the factual error that 'in Ottawa and London there was no significant difference between the A1 and A2 milk groups.'

Students of logic or debating may recognise in the paragraph above more than a hint of what is known as an 'appeal to authority' whereby an argument relies on its source (for example, 'distinguished international panel of authors' and 'experienced researchers') rather than on genuine logic.

Truswell then moved on to denigrate the heart-disease epidemiology of Laugesen and Elliott. He said that 'the use of average dietary consumption between countries against CHD [coronary heart disease] incidence has been abandoned by all serious researchers.' Students of logic will immediately recognise this as an *ad hominem* argument, albeit sophisticated, where Truswell, to use an analogy, was attacking the man rather than the ball. The clear implication of Truswell's statement was that Laugesen and Elliott could not be serious researchers if they were using these methods. Well, in that case why do peer-reviewed scientific journals still publish these studies? Let's be very clear: they remain a *very* important part of epidemiology when properly conducted.

Truswell criticises the heart-disease trial with rabbits on the grounds of an 'unsuitable animal model' and then again as 'not a realistic model for human atherosclerosis'. This is a fascinating claim and a magnificent way of brushing aside these results. A quick search of the PubMed database produced:

- 8073 citations of papers containing the words 'rabbits', 'heart', and 'disease';
- 3767 citations of papers containing the words 'rabbits' and 'atherosclerosis';
- 2936 citations of papers containing the words 'rabbits', 'ischaemic' and 'heart';
- 601 citations of papers containing the words 'rabbits' and 'atheroma'; and
- 337 citations of papers containing the words 'rabbits' and 'statins'.

So if rabbits are an unsuitable animal model for investigating heart disease how is it that so many researchers are wasting time and money studying them?

Truswell also criticised Professor Julie Campbell's work because, he claimed, 'measurements of the aortic fatty streaks were not made blind to the diet group.' However, I have checked this with Professor Campbell, and she tells me that the diet codes were not broken until all measurements were complete. In other words, the measurements *were* made without the scientists doing the measurements knowing which animals received which diets.

In his 2006 response in the *EJCN* to my own *EJCN* letter, Truswell referred to the Chin-Dusting *et al* (2006) paper that investigated the short-term cardiovascular response to A1 beta-casein. He described this paper as a 'large study' involving 24 subjects. Whether 24 people is a large study is debatable, but in fact the trial involved even fewer people: six men and nine women! He also failed to mention that this short-term trial reported diet confounding, with up to 20% A1 beta-casein in the supposed A2 beta-casein diet. In addition, the participants were still drinking normal milk in a range of dairy products as well as the supplementary diets of the trial.

Interestingly, one of Truswell's arguments against the rabbit trial (which showed heart disease with A1 beta-casein) was that the trial was short-term, whereas in humans heart disease is a chronic disease that develops over decades. (An alternative perspective is that it is in fact very impressive that the results did show up so quickly in these rabbits.) Yet suddenly he is using the similarly short-term, flawed Chin-Dusting trial, which failed to measure a difference, to buttress his own arguments!

Basically Truswell ignored the evidence in relation to autism and schizophrenia. In his 2006 response he said that he was aware of Cade's work but thought that the result was not 'clear cut'. He also said that he had 'not yet seen clear evidence that this peptide [BCM7] is released and active in humans *in vivo*'. I imagine that would raise the eyebrows of Cade, Reichelt and others. Readers may like to look again at this evidence in Chapter 8.

I could continue in similar vein, but I think the message is already clear. There were other errors in Truswell's logic, including faulty reasoning based on a misunderstanding of the statistical concept of standard error of a regression coefficient. (I subsequently addressed that issue in my letter published in March 2006 in the *EJCN*.)

So we can move on from the Truswell counter-attack. But the ongoing controversy in relation to A1 beta-casein raises another pertinent question. If the evidence is apparently so convincing, and the counter-evidence apparently so weak, then why is the issue still controversial?

At least part of the answer would seem to be that although many individual pieces of the puzzle are not particularly controversial, the whole story has not previously been brought together. Very few people have been looking for the big picture, and of course there have also been powerful forces that would prefer the status quo to remain. It has been far too complex an issue to deal with via the news media, although programmes such as 'White Mischief' on Australian television tried hard to present at least part of the story.

The reality is that many discoveries that threaten existing medical beliefs and practices take years to gain acceptance. An outstanding example of this is the discovery by Australian Nobel Prize winners Dr Robin Warren and Professor Barry Marshall that nearly all duodenal ulcers and 80% of stomach ulcers are caused by a bacterium that is now called *Helicobacter pylori*. Robin Warren made the key discovery back in 1979 that people with gastric ulcers also had unidentified bacteria in their stomachs. (Actually, the presence of bacteria in the stomachs of ulcer sufferers had first been noticed about 100 years earlier, but no-one thought it was important.) By 1984 Robin Warren and Barry Marshall had a key publication about this in the *Lancet*. Barry Marshall, much to the distress of his wife, even deliberately infected himself with *Helicobacter* to demonstrate cause and effect. Although disbelieving scientific reviewers had delayed its publication, by the mid-1980s this information was all in the public arena. Even I, a non-medico but someone who is always interested in new discoveries, was aware of it by 1986. But the medical profession resisted this new information that would turn existing medical practice on its head, and many years passed before antibiotics became the standard treatment of stomach and duodenal ulcers. As late as 2000 their work was still being described as 'controversial'. And it was only in 2005 that Warren and Marshall received the Nobel Prize for their work. This fascinating story is widely available on the internet.

Professor Peter Doherty is another Australian Nobel laureate who had to work hard to get full acknowledgement of his ideas. The paper on immunology that led to his Nobel Prize in 1996 was published in *Nature* way back in 1974. Peter Doherty has made the observation that to be a Nobel Prize winner a key criterion is to be long-lived. His message was not that most Nobel prizes require a lifetime's work; in fact scientists usually make their path-breaking discoveries quite early in life. But it can take a very long time to get acceptance of those ideas.

Some people have suggested to me that the work of people like Bob Elliott, Corran McLachlan, Robert Cade and Kalle Reichelt is of Nobel

Prize standard. I agree. But already it is too late for Corran McLachlan, as these prizes are never awarded posthumously. And there won't be any prizes while there is controversy.

If you want to find another analogy, you only have to think of the business and health battles that have swirled around cigarettes and smoking for the last 50 years despite the mountain of evidence.

Coming back to the milk devil itself, there are, of course, still lots of things we do not know. And the path of knowledge is never straight. We do not know for sure whether BCM7 is likely to be a problem in cheese. The epidemiological and theoretical evidence suggests it may not be a problem, or at least less of a problem, but we really don't know. Similarly, whether the biochemical processes involved in making yoghurt result in either more or less BCM7 being released has yet to be investigated. And it is unknown whether or not there is an increased release of BCM7 caused by the typical heat processes that many ice-cream makers use. But it is at least a possibility.

So now it is time for milk consumers to make up their own minds. Does it make sense that we should convert our dairy herds back to the original A2 type? And does it make sense for consumers to give preference to A2 milk products?

Consumers who live in cities or towns where A2 milk is currently sold are fortunate that they can make their own choices. But this is only the case if they can get access to good information. And for consumers who live in places where A2 milk is not available, then only consumer lobbying is likely to change that situation. Of course, if the New Zealand Government were to accept Professor Boyd Swinburn's recommendation in his report to the NZFSA that 'appropriate Government agencies have a responsibility to communicate the current state of evidence to the public' then the task would be much easier.

My hope is that this book might help people make informed decisions. I also hope this book might help people to think about the complex forces that influence the information and choices that are available to us. Are we satisfied with the way the system works? You be the judge.

NOTES

1 These papers are listed in the Industry, Marketing and Overview section of the Bibliography.

2 See Heart Disease section of Bibliography.

POSTSCRIPT

Since *Devil in the Milk* was first published in New Zealand in September 2007, the story has moved on considerably. The purpose of this postscript is therefore to update events through to October 2010, recognising that it will continue to be an ongoing story, and only time will allow some events to be seen in their appropriate context. Essentially, there are three parts to the ongoing story. The first is about the politics of milk and health, how information is communicated, and market responses. The second is about what is quietly happening 'behind the scenes' to dairy herds at a national and international level. The third is about new science that is providing exciting new information. All three parts of the ongoing story are important to an overall understanding.

Politics, the media and commerce

Publication of *Devil in the Milk* was certainly controversial. When the New Zealand and Australian edition of the book came out in September 2007 (the American edition from Chelsea Green was first published in 2009) there was an immediate media reaction. I found myself doing more than 40 radio and television interviews within the first week in both New Zealand and Australia. However, the response varied in each country.

In Australia, I was interviewed by Helen Wellings on Channel Seven's programme 'Today Tonight'. This programme was particularly important in bringing the 'A2 issue' to the attention of a major segment of the population. It was only a brief segment of about six minutes, and so it could not explore many of the issues, but it was seen by millions. I also gave a six-minute commentary for ABC Radio National in Australia, which was played at prime time in the evening and again in the morning. There was no interviewer; the producer simply gave me six minutes in which to say what I wanted. According to an A2 Corporation information release to the Stock Exchange, the impact of my book though the publicity that it generated was closely linked to more than doubling of the sales of A2 milk across Australia within a very short time. Sales have continued to grow, and have more than doubled again. By mid 2009, A2 milk was available in almost all Australian supermarkets right across Australia. Also, as of April 2010, A2 yoghurt became available under the Jalna brand. However, A2 milk in Australia remains a niche product, albeit now profitable, selling at a significant premium over other branded milks.

The initial response at the time of publication from Fonterra, headquartered in New Zealand, was to say nothing. This was exactly what I expected. Three weeks before publication, the Fonterra CEO had asked me in a telephone conversation to delay the release of the book for six months so they could undertake an internal review, but by that late stage I was neither able nor willing to accommodate them. (The reason they knew the book was coming was because I had told them.) So the internal advice of their public relations people was to say nothing and hope the controversy would blow over.

In contrast, the New Zealand Food Safety Authority (NZFSA) came out with all guns blazing. They claimed that there was nothing new in the book, but then had to admit that they had not had time to read it. On New Zealand national television (TV One), NZFSA spokesperson Carole Inkster and I were interviewed together in a live interview, Inkster from Wellington and me from Christchurch. Inkster claimed that if there had been anything new since the Swinburn review, Professor Swinburn would have advised them. That was easy to refute. I said that I had rung Professor Swinburn in Australia some three days earlier, and he had confirmed to me that he had not been working in this field for three years. Inkster also repeated the line that the Swinburn review had found that all milk was safe. I pointed out that nowhere in his report had Professor Swinburn said that all milk was safe.

At that time the television producer was unable to make contact with Professor Swinburn, who was by then on a working trip to Samoa, but Radio New Zealand National did manage to interview him from Samoa two days later. Professor Swinburn confirmed that he had never used those words, and also that he was very frustrated with the way that NZFSA had managed the release of his report. He made it clear that there were important health issues involved. He also defended my own integrity, which was nice to hear.

The NZFSA was unable to argue against the substance of what I wrote, but they were embarrassed by what I had exposed. So instead they attacked me personally (my qualifications to write on such matters), the format of the book (paperback), and also my publisher (non-scientific). Subsequently, the Minister of Food Safety at that time, Lianne Dalziel, apologised to me in writing for the manner of the attack by the NZFSA bureaucrats. She also repeated that apology when we met more recently at a social event.

There was also an attack in the media from a group of scientists from the University of Otago, led by Professor Jim Mann. Professor Mann is mentioned in several places in *Devil in the Milk* and at various times he was an adviser to Fonterra. Professor Mann did his credibility little good by criticising my book but then admitting that he too had not read it and was too busy. 'I haven't read his book and I'm not going to. I have better things to do with my life. I have got too much to do'.[1] However, he had found the time to check my publication record in relation to medical science, which he had found wanting.

In Chapters 3, 6, 11 and 13 of this book I make extensive mention of Professor Stewart Truswell from Sydney University. Professor Truswell confirmed in writing in the New Zealand Dairy Exporter (December 2007) that he had been a paid consultant of Fonterra in relation to A1 and A2 beta-casein. There is, of course, nothing wrong with being a consultant for Fonterra. However, some of us would have liked this disclosure made a lot earlier.

Another scientist from Otago who criticised the book in the general media (print and radio) was Dr Tony Merriman. Dr Merriman is a researcher investigating the genetic aspects of Type 1 diabetes. His criticism related specifically to the epidemiological link between Type 1 diabetes and intake of A1 beta-casein. He put forward the alternative hypothesis that the between-country differences in Type 1 diabetes can be explained by latitudinal effects influencing exposure to UV light and subsequent impact on Vitamin D synthesis. It is indeed true that there is a cross-correlation between latitude and intake of A1 beta-casein, and this was discussed in Chapter 5. This is because many of the countries with high intake of A1 beta-casein are also high-latitude countries. But there are plenty of exceptions. And the Laugesen and Elliott evidence shows that the explanatory power of latitude in relation to Type 1 diabetes is only half that of A1 beta-casein.[2] In the case of sunlight there was no meaningful relationship at all (M. Laugesen, personal communication).

So it is possible that the modest latitude correlation is being dragged along by its association with A1 beta-casein, but the evidence does not support the converse notion that the strong A1 beta-casein relationship can be explained by the modest latitudinal relationship.

What I do accept is that Vitamin D may well be part of the overall story on Type 1 diabetes. I made very clear in the concluding paragraphs of Chapter 7 that causation of Type 1 diabetes is almost certainly multifactorial. It is only when a number of factors line up together that the disease manifests itself. There is evidence that Type 1 diabetes typically reaches the clinical stage during winter, when UV radiation is lowest (although the development of the disease occurs over a much longer period), and there is also emerging evidence that those with Type 1 diabetes may have lower circulating Vitamin D levels (although there are very interesting issues about what may be causing the low Vitamin D levels). Indeed, low blood levels of Vitamin D may be associated with a broad range of health conditions including parathyroid disease, kidney disease, intestinal cancers and prostate cancers. Personally, I find the evidence for this to be strong. But what I do say very strongly is that neither latitude nor sunlight exposure can be used to explain away the relationship that exists between Type 1 diabetes incidence and intake of A1 beta-casein.

Some weeks following publication of my book, I released further information obtained under the Official Information Act as to how NZFSA dealt with the Swinburn review.[3] It had taken me some time to obtain this information (NZFSA had delayed releasing it to me), and so it was not in the first edition of this book. Despite the omission of key information in the released documentation that was 'whited out' on the grounds of confidentiality, the material was sufficiently embarrassing that NZFSA had to do something. They were also put under pressure by Christchurch journalist Paul Gorman who wrote a series of articles in *The Press* exposing their inconsistencies, and for which Gorman won a major media award. So NZFSA announced that they would be calling in an external consultant to review NZFSA risk-management procedures, including specific consideration as to how these procedures were applied to the issue of A1 and A2 milk. Remarkably, the NZFSA CEO, Andrew McKenzie, said on Radio New Zealand National that the aim was 'to bury the issue once and for all' and that the key issue was to demonstrate the integrity of the NZFSA. Not surprisingly, those comments led to some raised eyebrows.

The review was undertaken by Dr Stuart Slorach from Sweden.

Although external to the NZFSA, his investigations could hardly be called independent. He visited New Zealand and made a hurried visit to me in Christchurch (he could spare less than one hour) and also to Auckland. In Christchurch he was accompanied by the Chief Scientist for NZFSA and in Auckland by the CEO Andrew McKenzie. When his report came out in May 2008, it suggested many ways in which NZFSA could be improved. But the release of the report and the associated media conference were carefully stage-managed by NZFSA. The key statements in regard to A1 beta-casein were deeply buried on page 41 of the report.

> The assertion that *'there is no safety issue with either type of milk'* can be interpreted in different ways. If it is interpreted, as some do, as meaning that there is no scientific debate about possible negative health effects of A1 milk, it is not correct and is also contradicted by the quotes from Swinburn's report given lower down in the same media release. According to NZFSA, the phrase *'there is no safety issue with either type of milk'* was intended to provide the public with assurance that their choice to use either (A1 or A2) milk product was not going to result in the safety issues that are otherwise associated with unsafe food, such as sickness or hospitalisation.

What a remarkable statement! Suddenly NZFSA were telling Dr Slorach that they were never referring to the negative health effects discussed in my book, but to other issues associated with unsafe food! But of course this contradicts much of what they had been saying in public.

Ironically, over the next two years, if any readers were to seek out information on this issue on the NZFSA website (www.nzfsa.govt.nz), they would easily find information critical of me in NZFSA's own press releases. They would get to this information very quickly from the home page by clicking on 'A1 and A2 milk'. But they would have struggled to find Dr Slorach's report except by scrolling down and eventually finding it at the bottom via a 'related link'. Originally, Dr Slorach's report could not be found there at all, but following my remonstrations to the Food Safety Minister Lianne Dalziel, NZFSA did make it available, even if deeply buried. The message I took from this was that bureaucrats have many ways to defend their public reputations.

More recently, the NZFSA website has been reorganised, but a site search using my name will quickly lead to critical material about me, and a search on 'Slorach' will lead to the Slorach Report.

Since the publication of my book I have spoken to many medical and scientific groups both in New Zealand and Australia. One of the most interesting requests was to present the closing plenary paper to the International Diabetes Federation (IDF) Western Pacific Congress.[4] This was set up as a forum, with Professors Boyd Swinburn and Bob Elliott as commentators on my paper. Both Swinburn and Elliott were strongly supportive, but the co-chair, Professor Len Harrison from Australia, gave a summing up that was much more cautious, perhaps even negative. The original plan had been to have commentators who would give both positive and negative commentary, but those asked to speak in the negative had pulled out. So it was disappointing when the co-chair took on that role. Professor Harrison had taken a similar stance when interviewed for the Four Corners White Mischief programme on Australian TV some years previously.[5]

Although aspects of the IDF Diabetes presentation were frustrating, there was some good that came out of it. The informal discussions that were held led to Professor Swinburn, whom NZFSA had falsely claimed as supporting their 'all milk is safe' stance, now taking a stronger public position. He sent an open letter to the New Zealand media, and addressed to all farmers, stating that the time to shift their herds to A2 was 'right now'. He clarified his position by saying that, although in his opinion there was still no final proof, the potential benefits to public health were sufficiently strong, and the costs so small, that it should be done.

In some ways Professor Swinburn's position was not all that different to back in 2004 when, in private correspondence with NZFSA (which I obtained through the Official Information Act) and in remonstrating with them as to how they were handling his report, he had said:

> . . . if I had a child with Type 1 diabetes and was due to have another and I could easily obtain and afford A2 milk or formula, I would certainly use it for the next child because the cost/benefit is low because of the potentially very large benefit of preventing Type 1 diabetes.

Some people have asked me why Professor Swinburn did not go public a lot earlier. My response is that he was in a difficult position. He had undertaken the study for NZFSA under contract, and therefore they owned the report. He chose initially to remonstrate with them in private rather than in public. I admire him greatly for subsequently going public.

Given my professional position within agribusiness, I regularly come into contact with various Fonterra directors and senior management. However, I have been unable to convince them to engage with the issue. They continue to take the advice of Fonterra's Chief Scientist Jeremy Hill, who features so prominently within my book, that the issue has no substance. It seems to me that none of the directors or top level management are willing to engage on the issue because they lack confidence in their own ability to read and understand the science. So, they simply rely on Fonterra's scientific leader. That in itself is a fundamental flaw within Fonterra's governance and management.

In terms of industry politics and the 'PR game', the publication in January 2009 of a European Food Safety (EFSA) Scientific Report titled 'Review of the potential health impact on ß-casomorphins and related peptides' was a major win for those opposing the A2 issue. The background to this report was that NZFSA, under instructions from the NZ Government, and in addition to commissioning Dr Slorach to look at their procedures, had asked EFSA to review the substantive scientific issues around the A1/A2 milk debate. This led to EFSA deciding to undertake its own review, which was completed on 29 January 2009.[6] They concluded:

> Based on the present review of available scientific literature, a cause-effect relationship between the oral intake of BCM7 or related peptides and aetiology or course of any suggested non-communicable diseases cannot be established.

At a political level, this outcome was a major blow to the A2 cause. It has been used to good effect by those who want to bury the issue (i.e. the mainstream dairy industry). But the finding was an inevitable outcome of how EFSA defined the evidential requirement. To determine cause-effect using their criteria, there would have needed to be human clinical trials which showed a clear quantitative relationship between the intake of BCM7 and the risk for individuals. That information does not exist. And if it did exist it would almost certainly vary for different individuals, given the apparent link with 'leaky gut'. Of course there is strong evidence at the population level, but EFSA chose for its own reasons to not place weight on that evidence.

On reading the EFSA report I was puzzled by the negativity. In particular, I found myself reading in the report the same arguments made by the mainstream dairy industry that I have already presented in *Devil in the Milk*. I found that they were questioning rabbits as a suitable model (I discussed that in Chapter 13). I also found they were using the FAD trial (discussed in detail in Chapter 6) without any acknowledgement of the contamination issue. But clearly at least some people in EFSA should have known of the issue, given that Food Safety Minister Lianne Dalziel told me that she received a 'yes' to her explicit question as to whether they had my book and were aware of the arguments therein. They were also using the strongly flawed Caerphilly cohort data (discussed in Chapter 3) as contradictory information to the A2 hypothesis. They essentially ignored the Laugesen and Elliot epidemiology on the grounds that such studies supposedly prove nothing. They used the elementary argument that ecological (i.e. between-country) studies are liable to find false associations on account of lifestyle factors. But they ignored the fact that the A1/A2 epidemiology is restricted to developed country comparisons and hence to developed country lifestyles. They also ignored the painstaking but unsuccessful search by Laugesen and Elliott for alternative factors that could have been confounding. It seemed to me that EFSA knew the answers they wanted from the outset.

So I set to work to find out a little more about the eight authors. On searching databases I found that five could be classed as dairy scientists with strengths in biochemistry. Another two were trained in veterinary faculties and now specialise in toxicity and pharmacology. The remaining one is a human nutrition professor from Iceland (Professor Thorsdottir) who is listed in *Devil in the Milk* as a co-author of papers suggesting that A1 beta casein is indeed a risk factor in Type 1 diabetes. Where were the human health experts in heart disease, diabetes and autism? Where were the experts on food intolerances and leaky gut? Where were the medical experts in population health studies and epidemiology? I was no longer quite so puzzled as to the content and tone of the report.

Indeed the EFSA outcome was exactly what some people had been warning me. If the EFSA report had found against A1 beta-casein, even as something that was uncertain, then the worldwide implications for the milk industry could have been both enormous and unfortunate. Parts of the media would inevitably have interpreted it as a finding against all milk rather than a component that can be easily bred out of our dairy herds. And a positive finding would have led to a formal investigation to determine maximum safe intakes. So perhaps the outcome was predestined.

In the days following the release of the report, the media sought Professor Boyd Swinburn's latest opinion. He stated that in his view A2 remained the safe option, and that none of the science was refuted. He also said that the evidential barrier was very high and the terms of reference narrow. Given those narrow terms of reference, he said that the conclusions might be defensible but not helpful. That also summed up my perspective.

Nevertheless, the EFSA report did provide a very valuable crutch for the dairy industry in both New Zealand and Australia. I know of no-one apart from one scientist who has actually read the full report, but in terms of letting industry off the hook, at least in the short term, it has been very effective. Both Dairy Australia and Fonterra have used it to good effect as a publicity weapon. Dairy Australia has even gone further by making claims such as "There is no good scientific evidence that A2 milk is any different to A1 milk".[7]

In April 2010 there was further publicity in Australia as a result of a programme on the ABC 7.30 report for which I was interviewed. I considered the programme to be disappointing. Important and impressive interview material by Professor Boyd Swinburn was cut at the last moment, although the extended version with Swinburn's comments included is still (October 2010) available on the ABC website.[8] Also, a number of incorrect statements from the opposing side went unchallenged. The mainstream industry tried to portray the 'A2 issue' as a marketing gimmick that lacked scientific evidence. Nevertheless, the publicity did lead to a further boost to A2 milk sales across Australia.

Outside of Australia, progress has been slower. In New Zealand, A2 milk is available through many Countdown, Woolworths and Fresh Choice supermarkets. But unlike Australia, there is almost no publicity. In the United States, A2 milk was available for a period in Hy-Vee supermarkets in seven Midwest States. However, in December 2008 the A2 Milk Company announced they were withdrawing product from sale pending a re-branding and re-launch on a broader scale across the US. To date that has not occurred. The evidence is clear that it is hard to market a product where the issues are complex, where there are constraints on the promotion of that message, and where consumers remain ignorant or confused about the issues.

In July 2010, A2 Corporation confirmed that it was buying out its Australian joint venture partner Freedom Nutritional Products (FNP), with FNP then becoming a 25% equity partner within A2 Corporation.

Subsequently, FNP's Managing Director and CEO, Geoffrey Babidge, became Managing Director of A2 Corporation. In addition, in October 2010, A2 Corporation made a further announcement that it had bought out its joint venture partner Ideasphere in the USA in return for a small placement of A2 Corporation shares with Ideasphere. The inference is that A2 Corporation is moving into pro-active mode internationally.

Converting the national herds

There is a lot of ongoing confusion as to exactly what is meant by 'A2 milk'. In terms of the commercial product, currently only available in New Zealand and Australia, it is the product labelled and trademarked as 'a2 Milk'. This milk comes from herds which are comprised totally of cows that produce only A2 beta-casein and not A1 beta-casein. However, all herds contain some cows that produce A2 beta-casein ('A2 cows'), plus other cows that produce a mix of A1 and A2 beta-casein, plus other cows that produce only the A1 variant of beta-casein. From a public health perspective, progress can be made by increasing the number of A2 cows in the national herds, and this can be done, over time, simply by using A2 bulls.

To some extent this is occurring, particularly in New Zealand. In part this is because some farmers are purposely using only A2 semen. (There has been sufficient publicity that almost every dairy farmer in New Zealand must be aware of the issue.) It is also because a particularly high proportion of the top New Zealand bulls are homozygous A2 (i.e. carry two copies of the A2 variant of the beta-casein gene). Given that almost all of the bulls in New Zealand are genetically tested for A2 status, this information is publicly available. However, I have more work to do, using data from the breeding companies as to the number of artificial inseminations from each bull, to document exactly what is happening. At this stage my best estimate is that the proportion of the beta-casein in New Zealand milk that is A2 has been increasing since about Year 2000 at about 1.5% per annum. Whereas in the late 1990s it would have been about 50% A1 and 50% A2, I believe it is now, in 2010, closer to 35% A1 and 65% A2. I am confident that the A2 level is going to continue to rise at about 2% per annum through to 2012, given the lag between time of mating and subsequent arrival of the progeny in the milking herd. So it may not be too long before New Zealand is up to the levels that are found in some of the southern European countries.

In Australia there is probably a similar but smaller drift occurring.

However, many farmers in Australia are less aware of the issue than New Zealand farmers. They have been fed information by Dairy Australia that it is a non-issue. But perusal of the bull semen catalogues indicates a similar preponderance of A2 bulls and so some serendipity will be occurring.

Many people continue to tell me that this unannounced drift to A2 in New Zealand, and perhaps the smaller drift in Australia, has to be a conspiracy, but I can see no evidence for that. It is genuine serendipity caused by A2 bulls ranking highly for productive traits. This is linked to the criteria of the New Zealand national breeding system which favours medium liveweight animals with a high percentage of protein in their milk. These animals tend to by homozygous A2 through chance. But there is a huge irony. Fonterra continues to tell the world dairy community that A1 beta-casein is a non-issue, and I keep hearing this from dairy companies overseas as far afield as Mexico to Sweden. So no countries apart from New Zealand, and to a lesser extent Australia, are doing anything about it in terms of their mainstream national herds.

In the United States some individual producers are now converting their herds. This is particularly the case with the Guernsey breed, which are in any case naturally very high in A2. As from 2010, licensed testing of cows has also been available through the University of California at Davis.

New science

DPP4 First of all, I need to explain what I now regard as an omission from the first edition of *Devil in the Milk*. I should have written about the enzyme dipeptidyl peptidase4, commonly abbreviated to DPP4. It is this enzyme which breaks down BCM7. Within the digestive system, this enzyme is only found attached to epithelial cells in the lining of the stomach and intestines. On the one hand this can be used to explain why, for people with properly functioning digestive systems, the BCM7 should not get through except in possibly very minor quantities into the blood. But it also provides an explanation why, for those who have an impaired digestive system with damaged epithelial cells (a 'leaky gut'), the BCM7 can sneak through. That potentially includes all those people with undiagnosed or untreated stomach ulcers, ulcerative colitis, Crohns, and untreated sufferes of Coeliac disease. It can also include those who have been on antibiotics, or are subject to various stress factors. I am also now aware, but was not when I wrote the first edition, that there is a considerable body of evidence showing that genetic susceptibility to Type 1 diabetes is linked to susceptible people having a naturally leaky gut. So this would seem to be one more piece of the jigsaw.

Much of the information about DPP4 has been known for quite some time. However, increased understanding is now developing about how BCM7 crosses what is known as the caco-2 monolayer (between the digestive system and the circulatory system) in the presence of DPP4. This work is coming out of Poland, with Malgorzata Iwan the lead author of a 2008 paper in the journal Peptides. Indeed the group to which Iwan belongs has been particularly active in investigating the biochemistry of both human and bovine BCM7 and also linking it to allergies. Their work can be found readily by searching the Pubmed public access electronic database (www.ncbi.nlm.nih.gov/sites/entrez) and searching on the word 'casomorphin'.

Natalya Kost Perhaps the most exciting recent work has come from a Russian group of 12 scientists from four leading research institutions, and funded by the Russian Foundation for Basic Research. (In scientific circles, 'basic' means 'fundamental' or 'non commercial'). It is published in the international journal *Peptides*, with Natalya Kost as the lead author.[9] The Russians have been steadily building up knowledge on BCM7 for quite some years, but it is only now that they have started publishing in English.

Natalya Kost and colleagues have made three complementary breakthroughs. First, they have successfully developed tests for measuring BCM7 in the blood. This might seem very simple, but blood is a complex substance, and until now it has only been possible to measure BCM7 in urine and digestive fluids. Being able to test for BCM7 in the blood will be a huge step forward for subsequent research. Second, the Russians have shown that babies fed formula milk do indeed absorb BCM7 into their blood. This absorption is exactly what would be expected on theoretical grounds, given the permeability of babies' digestive systems, but it is a huge step to go from theory to empirical evidence.

However, the Russians have gone much further than that. They have shown that some of the babies can eliminate the BCM7 rapidly from their systems (either through metabolising or excreting it), but that other babies retain it in the bloodstream. Then comes the final blow. Those babies who are unable to rapidly breakdown and excrete the BCM7 from their systems are at very high risk of delayed psychomotor development.

In other words, development of the neurological links from brain to muscles is delayed. The Russians found in their study that 30% of the babies fed formula had developmental delay whereas only 3% of breast fed babies were in that category.

There is a lot more of importance in the Russian paper. For example, they have shown that the human form of BCM7 (which is actually considerably different in its biochemical structure to the bovine form found in A1 milk and which is found only in breast milk) is actually a good casomorphin, at least in small quantities, that enhances psychomotor development and works best in those children who don't break it down quickly. It is only the bovine form, released in large quantities from A1 cows, that is the 'devil'.

When history looks back on the saga of A1 beta-casein and the 'milk devil' I think the verdict will be that this Kost *et al* paper is the most significant breakthrough for at least five years. It is not only the results themselves, but that the Russians have given major new insights which others can now follow up. For example, the insight that it is not just a case of whether the BCM7 is absorbed, but also whether or not the individual has the ability to rapidly metabolise and excrete the little devil, will open the door to new research pathways.

Of course much of the mainstream industry is attempting to downplay this research. Dairy Australia, when it became aware of this research, was quick to emphasise the earlier and greatly flawed EFSA report which attempted to hose down the A1 milk issue. The New Zealand Food Safety Authority said that the Russian research was just one paper and that the results needed confirmation. Others have tried to downplay it because it has come from Russia. But the bell is now tolling. This is not just a report by some mad scientist with a 'bee in his bonnet'. It is a peer reviewed paper in an international journal by 12 scientists from four leading research institutions, with funding from the Russian Foundation for Basic Research. All praise to the Russians.

Alexandra Steinerova Another stream of new research has emerged from the Czech Republic. For more than 10 years, Alexandra Steinerova and colleagues have been untangling the causes of oxidative stress in infants. It is a fascinating story of how one investigation leads to another; of how BCM7 and A1 beta-casein were subsequently implicated; and then how causation has been subsequently demonstrated.

The research is important because oxidative LDL (caused by oxidative stress) and antibodies thereto, are key risk factors and indicators of heart disease. They are also important indicators of Alzheimer's disease.

Most people associate heart disease with easily measured cholesterol. But amongst researchers, oxidised LDL is much more important because it is this substance that makes arteries sticky and leads to formation of plaque.

The initial work of Steinerova and colleagues showed that, during the first few months of age, some babies have increasing antibodies to oxidised LDL, whereas others have declining values relative to levels at birth. In their first paper, in 1999, Steinerova and colleagues were unable to explain the findings.

Then in 2001, they reported that further work had shown that it was the babies on milk formula who had the increasing levels, and the breast-fed babies were the ones with declining levels. In fact, by three months of age the formula fed babies had almost 50 times the antibodies to oxidised LDL of the breast-fed babies. They offered no hypothesis as to which component(s) within milk formula might be causing this.

In 2004, Steinerova and her colleagues reported in the journal *Atherosclerosis* that they were by then hypothesising that it was caused by BCM7 from A1 beta-casein. I mentioned this in the first edition of *Devil in the Milk*, but at that stage it seemed to me that it was still just a hypothesis, although supported by earlier work by French scientists Torreilles and Guerin who had shown in the test tube that BCM7 does indeed oxidise LDL. Accordingly, at that time I wrote (p83): "this is an evolving story, with quite a lot known, but still much more to be discovered".

Steinerova and colleagues published more evidence in 2006, but this was in a Czech medical journal (*CS.Pediatrie*)[10] and was not widely available to English-speaking people. It was only when Steinerova and colleagues presented a paper in the United States at the XV International Symposium on Atherosclerosis in 2009 that the strength of their evidence became apparent. They now have new data not only confirming their original results (although this time the difference in oxidised LDL in formula-fed infants was only 18 times that in the breast-fed babies), but also now showing that the formula-fed babies had very high antibodies to BCM7 and A1 beta-casein, whereas breast-fed did not. Equally important, the antibodies to A2 beta-casein were much lower.

Arguably, there was still a weakness in the argument. These results were based on what is called epidemiology. This epidemiology clearly showed there was an association between A1 beta-casein and BCM7 on the one hand, and high levels of oxidative stress. And the statistical analysis showed that this was highly unlikely to be due to chance. But for those people who want proof rather than just exceptionally strong evidence, there was still no clinical trial. Where was the direct trial comparing A1 and A2 beta-casein?

In fact, Steinerova and colleagues do have an answer to that. In their 2006 paper in the journal *CS.Pediatrie* they reported that piglets fed A1 beta-casein had much higher and statistically significant levels of antibodies to oxidised LDL than did those fed A2 beta-casein. So yes, they have established what is known as 'cause and effect'.

So, are there any remaining weaknesses in this line of work from the Czech Republic? Those who wish to deny the links between BCM7 and health (and there are plenty of those people associated with the international milk industry) will make three claims. The first is that the trial was with pigs and not with humans. That is true. However, the combination of the human epidemiology and the animal results points only in one direction. The second criticism is that Steinerova has not published her recent work in top quality western journals, but instead she has published in a peer reviewed Czech language medical journal. Yes, that too is true. And until she does publish all of this work in English it will not receive the full attention that it deserves. The third criticism will probably be that the pigs when slaughtered at six months of age did not have visible heart disease. That too is true; but that is not surprising, for heart disease takes a long time to build up.

The bottom line is that Steinerova's work provides chilling support to the prior body of heart disease evidence, undertaken by researchers such as McLachlan, Laugesen and Elliott, Briggs, and Campbell, which I reported in the first edition of *Devil in the Milk*. It also dovetails nicely with the new research from Natalya Kost and colleagues showing that children fed formula not only absorb BCM7, but those who cannot then rapidly break it down or excrete it are likely to suffer developmental delay.

In the long run, Steinerova's work may prove to be much more important for adults than babies. It will be important for babies because oxidative stress is strongly linked to a range of health conditions in babies, particularly those born prematurely. But babies do not get heart disease, and it may well be that most of them outgrow the oxidative stress (although that is currently unknown, and it may well be a precursor of adult heart disease). However, if BCM7 causes oxidative stress and oxidised LDL in formula-fed babies (which Steinerova has clearly shown it does), then logic says it must also cause oxidative LDL in those adults who absorb BCM7 into the blood stream, i.e. those who have a leaky gut. So, here we now have a solid mechanism capable of explaining the link between BCM7 and heart disease. It ties in perfectly with the epidemiology, the rabbit work, and the evidence of Briggs about heart disease in ulcer sufferers on high milk diets.

Paul Whiteley Another field of research on which more data is emerging is the effect of casein-free gluten-free diets in relation to autism. In the past this work has been held back by the difficulty of implementing long term blind trials. In April 2010, Paul Whiteley and colleagues published data in the journal Nutritional Neuroscience, from what they call the ScanBrit study, of children on this diet for up to 2 years, where the investigators taking the measurements were blinded as to which children were on the diet and which were controls. (Not surprisingly, the parents could not be blinded.)[11] The evidence from the first year met predetermined statistical differences in outcomes such that the children on the control diet were, on ethical grounds, also offered the treatment in the second year. The evidence shows that the diet has benefits for some but not all children. And the trial design could not determine separate effects from gluten and casein. In my judgement, these results are generally supportive of the case against A1 beta-casein, but by themselves are not going to be a 'debate changer' in the way that the Russian and Czech work has potential to be.

Ivano De Noni Two recent papers by Ivano De Noni in the international journal *Food Chemistry* are particularly important.[12, 13] They are important not only because of what is said in these papers, but because of who is saying it. De Noni was one of the authors of the EFSA report which greatly downplayed the A2 issue. Yet here is De Noni publishing papers in the international peer reviewed literature that make some very important advances to knowledge.

De Noni's 2008 paper reports that BCM7 could not be found directly in either milk or infant formula. This is to be expected. However, once the milk and infant formula were digested in the laboratory, using enzymes and conditions as close as possible to those in the human digestive system, then BCM7 was indeed released from all commercial samples. It was also released from specially selected A1 samples but not from A2. De Noni is quite categorical (as indeed was the EFSA report) that BCM7 is not released from A2 under the conditions found in the human digestive system. Indeed he spends some time refuting a Polish study that, in contrast to a considerable number of other studies, apparently found small quantities of BCM7 released from A2 beta-casein. He points out weaknesses in their measuring techniques, and also points out that they were using conditions not found in the human gut. So here we have an 'establishment' milk scientist, and an acknowledged expert even by EFSA, saying that there is no doubt about the release of BCM7 from A1 beta-casein, and also no doubt that this does not occur from A2. Clearly this makes nonsense of the Dairy Australia statement referred to earlier in this Postscript that 'There is no good scientific evidence that A2 milk is any different to A1 milk'.[14]

Another informative finding from De Noni's 2008 paper is that BCM7 is also released from the B variant of beta-casein. This should come as no surprise given that B beta-casein is simply A1 beta-casein whose structure has been further influenced by a second mutation that changes an amino acid in another part of the protein. In other words, it has a histidine at position 67 so it is essentially part of the A1 family and hence it was always likely that it would release BCM7. However, I have previously received criticism on an American website for making this assumption, so it is nice that we now know this for sure. Somewhat surprisingly, De Noni actually found a higher release of BCM7 from the B than the A1. This suggests the second mutation affects the way the protein folds, and that this increases the release. B beta-casein is mainly found in Jersey cattle, but only in a minority of them.

Another hugely important finding of De Noni comes from his 2010 paper where he shows that BCM7 is released from the digestion of cheese and yoghurt. In the first edition of this book I said that we had no information about yoghurt, and also no convincing evidence about cheese. Well, that has now changed! De Noni also reports evidence that the release of BCM7 is not influenced by heat treatment. In other words, it does not matter how the milk is processed or what products it is turned into; if it comes from cows that produce A1 beta-casein then BCM7 will be released on digestion. No longer can this be a matter of debate; it is a matter of fact.

If there is any further debate as to the implications of De Noni's work, it will be that the amount of BCM7 released is insufficient to cause harm. However, the work of Kost and Steinerova, and also the previous work led by Sun, Cade and others, is demonstrating that small quantities getting through to the circulatory system on a regular basis do indeed have dramatic consequences. The amounts required to have an effect are considerably less than the amounts De Noni has reported as being released upon digestion of A1 beta-casein.

Observational evidence Another area where information continues to build up is in observational evidence, which some people dismissingly call 'anecdotal'. At one of my Australian talks to medical groups, Dr Mervyn Garrett, a specialist in food allergies and intolerances from the Gold Coast, stood up and said that he had successfully treated about 20 people with these problems by shifting them to A2 milk. He said he had a colleague in New South Wales who had successfully treated even more people than he had, but also had a few failures. Well, none of us have ever suggested that A1 milk is the only food that causes food-intolerance and allergy problems. In the last three years I have been approached by many people who say they can drink A2 milk after a lifetime of problems with ordinary milk. I have also had people tell me that they no longer have mucus problems that they had previously associated with milk. This is consistent with the link between casomorphins and mucins (the proteins in mucus) discussed in Chapter 9. It is difficult to be precise with numbers, but the evidence I see points to well over half the people who have previously been unable to tolerate 'ordinary' milk, because of conditions such as nausea, bloating and eczema, now finding that they are able to digest A2 milk. This is consistent with the notion that many people have been assumed to be lactose intolerant whereas it is really A1 beta-casein to which they are intolerant.

In summary, it seems to me that all of the new research published since the first edition of my book is pointing in the same direction. More pieces of the jigsaw have fallen into place. Also, the canvas on which that jigsaw lies has become bigger, with additional extensions and new insights. In particular, the findings of the teams led by Kost, Steinerova and De Noni, once combined together, are very powerful. There is also further ongoing research that I am aware of, and that I would love to talk about here, but until it is formally published I can say nothing.

A Final Comment

If there is one thing I have had reinforced since writing the first edition of *Devil in the Milk*, it is that the path of knowledge, and how that knowledge is communicated, is long and tortuous. Information, misinformation and vested interests get inextricably intertwined. Intellectual property rights to patents and trademarks, and how these might be interpreted in different jurisdictions, adds a further complication. In health and medical matters, truth will always win out in the long run, whatever that truth may be, but the journey can be very long. Despite all the emerging evidence, the beta-casein journey is far from over.

I plan to keep writing about further developments relating to A1 beta casein, A2 milk and BCM7 at http://keithwoodford.wordpress.com

KEITH WOODFORD
October 2010

NOTES

1 The Press, October 11 2007. www.stuff.co.nz/4233104a11.html

2 See Laugesen and Elliott (2003a) in Diabetes section of Bibliography

3 See Woodford, K (2007). 'The role of the NZFSA in investigating health issues concerning A1 and A2 milk.' Available at www.lincoln.ac.nz/story1057.html

4 The paper is available at www.lincoln.ac.nz/diabetes or from my own internet site at http://keithwoodford.wordpress.com

5 Australian Broadcasting Corporation. 2003. White Mischief. Available at www.abc.net.au/4corners/content/2003/transcripts/s820943.htm

6 Scientific Report of EFSA prepared by a DATEX Working group on the potential health impact of β-casomorphins and related peptides. EFSA Scientific Report (2009) 231,1-107. Available at http://www.efsa.europa.eu/EFSA/efsa_locale-1178620753812_home.htm

7 See http://www.weeklytimesnow.com.au/article/2010/04/27/179131_dairy.htm

8 Go to http://www.abc.net.au/reslib/201004/r544499_3184147.asx

9 Kost NV, et al. 2009. 'ß-casomorphin-7 in infants on different types of feeding and different levels of psychomotor development.' *Peptides* 2009 Oct; 30(10):1854-60.)

10 Steinerova, A, et al 2006. 'Does artificial suckling nutrition pose a risk of atherosclerosis at adult age?' Cesko *Slovenska Pediatrie* 61(9): 519-523

11 Whiteley, P et al 2010. 'The ScanBrit randomised, controlled, single-blind study of a gluten- and casein-free dietary intervention for children with autism spectrum disorders.' *Nutritional Neuroscience* 13(2):87-100.

12 De Noni, I 2008. 'Release of beta-casomorphins 5 and 7 during simulated gastro-intestinal digestion of bovine beta-casein variants and milk-based infant formulas.' *Food Chemistry* 110:897-903.

13 De Noni, I and Cattaneo, S. 2010. 'Occurrence of beta-casomorphins 5 and 7 in commercial dairy products and in their digests following in vitro simulated gastro-intestinal digestion.' *Food Chemistry* 119:560-566.

14 See http://www.weeklytimesnow.com.au/article/2010/04/27/179131_dairy.htm

BIBLIOGRAPHY

The websites and scientific papers listed below provide a starting point for people who want to read further on the issues discussed in this book. This is not the total scientific literature that is relevant to A1 beta-casein and the milk devil, but I have attempted to list everything that is of central importance based on what we currently know.

When scientists write scientific papers they are writing for a specialist audience and they use a lot of technical language. Accordingly a lot of these papers do not make for easy reading.

In some cases the important contents of the paper in relation to BCM7 and beta-casein are not evident from the title. In these cases I have added a brief indication of content at the end of the reference.

In contrast to scientific papers, website material is typically written for a general audience. However, anyone can place material on the web. Accordingly, I have only listed websites that I believe are authored by credible organisations. Of course anyone can obtain a great deal more information from a Google search but some of it may be total rubbish.

WEBSITES

A2 Corporation www.a2corporation.com The scientific reviews on this website are notable for their comprehensive literature bibliographies, and contain additional references not listed in this book.

A2 Milk Australia www.a2australia.com.au This is the website of the company that markets A2 milk in Australia.

Autism Network for Dietary Intervention www.autismndi.com This website is a good entry point for information related to diet and autism. It contains a mix of scientific information and anecdote.

Direct-MS www.direct-ms.com This website is a good entry point for information on nutrition and multiple sclerosis. It does not address the specific issue of A2 milk.

Harvard School of Public Health www.hsph.harvard.edu/nutritionsource/ This website is a good place to get an overview on issues about milk and human nutrition.

Keith Woodford's page on the Lincoln University website www.lincoln.ac.nz/story1057.html This contains information on A2 milk and many other agribusiness topics on which I write professionally.

PUBLISHED PAPERS

Milk and Casomorphins

Andiran F, Dayi S, Mete E. 2003. Cows milk consumption in constipation and anal fissure in infants and young children. *Journal of Paediatric Child Health* 39(5):329–331.

Becker A, Hempel G, Greksch G, Matthies H. 1990. Effects of beta-casomorphin derivatives on gastrointestinal transit in mice. *Biomedica Biochimica Acta* 49(110):1203–1207.

Brantl V, Teschemacher L. 1994. Beta casomorphins and related peptides. Weinheim: VCH.

Brantl V, Teschemacher H. 1979. A material with opioid activity in bovine milk and milk products. *Naunyn-Schmiedeberg's Archives of Pharmacology* 306(3):301–304. [An early publication reporting that compounds with opioid activity, which were resistant to peptidase digestion, were detected in 'certain batches of baby food, casein digest and cow milk in considerably varying amounts'.]

Chabance B, Marteau P, Rambaud JC, Migliore-Samour D, Boynard M, Perrotin P, Guillet R, Jolles P, Fiat AM. 1998. Casein peptides release and passage to the blood in humans during digestion of milk or yogurt. *Biochimie* 80(2):155–165. [Investigates the passage of peptides but not specifically BCM7.]

Claustre J, Toumi F, Trompette A, Jourdan G, Guignard H, Chayvialle JA, Plaisancie P. 2002. Effects of peptides derived from dietary proteins on mucus secretion in rat jejunum. *American Journal of Physiology, Gastrointestinal and Liver Physiology* 283(3):G521–528. [Found that BCM7 influenced intestinal secretions and that this was opioid-related.]

Defilippi C, Gomez E, Charlin V, Silva C. 1995. Inhibition of small intestine motility by casein: a role of beta casomorphins? *Nutrition* 119(6):751–754.

Dettmer K, Hanna D, Whetstone P, Hansen R, Hammock BD. 2007. Autism and urinary exogenous neuropeptides: development of an online SPE–HPLC–tandem mass spectrometry method to test the opioid excess theory. *Analytical and Bioanalytical Chemistry*. (Advance online publication May 2007. DOI 10.1007/s00216-007-1301-4).

Dubynin VA, Malinovskaya IV, Ivleva YA, Andreeva, LA, Kamenskii AA, Ashmarin IP. 2000. Delayed behavioral effects of beta-casomorphin-7 depend on age and gender of albino rats. *Bulletin of Experimental Biological Medicine* 130(11):1031–1034. [Links BCM7 to brain development in young rats.]

Hartwig A, Teschemacher H, Lehmann W, Gauly M, Erhadt G. 1997. Influence of genetic polymorphisms in bovine milk on the occurrence of bioactive peptides. In: *Milk Protein Polymorphism*, International Dairy Federation Special Publication 9702, pp 459–460, Brussels, Belgium.

Hedner J, Hedner T. 1987. Beta-casomorphins induce apnea and irregular breathing in adult rats and newborn rabbits. *Life Science* 41(20):2303–2312.

Henschen A, Lottspeich F, Brantl V, Teschemacher, H. 1979. Novel opioid peptides derived from casein (beta-casomorphins). II. Structure of active components from bovine casein peptone. *Hoppe Seylers Z Physiological Chemistry* 360(9): 1217–1224. [This was the first time BCM7 and its opioid characteristics were identified.]

Herrera-Marschitz M, Terenius L, Grehn L, Ungerstedt U. 1989. Rotational behaviour produced by intra nigral injections of bovine and human beta-casomorphin in rats. *Psychpharmacology (Berlin)* 99(3):357–361. [This paper found that bovine BCM5 was 10 times more potent than human BCM5, and also that it took 10 times as much naloxone to counteract the bovine BCM5 as it took to counteract the effects of morphine.]

Hill JP. 2003. The influence of consumption of A1 beta-casein on heart disease and Type 1 diabetes. *The New Zealand Medical Journal* 116(1169).

Huynh ML, Walsh BJ, Clarke AJ. 2006. A MS approach to determine the relative content of beta casein variants in milk. 31st Lorne Conference on Protein Structure and Function, Melbourne. [Available from Dr AJ Clarke, A2 Corporation.]

Iacono G, Cavataio F, Montalto G, Florena A, Tumminello M, Soresi M, Notarbartolo A, Carroccio A. 1998. Intolerance of cow's milk and chronic constipation in children. *New England Journal of Medicine* 339(16):1100–1104.

Jinsmaa Y, Yoshikawa M. 1999. Enzymatic release of neocasomorphin and beta-casomorphin from bovine beta-casein. *Peptides* 20(8):957–962.

Kim T-G, Choung J-J, Wallace RJ, Chamberlain DG. 2000. Effects of intra-abomasal infusion of beta-casomorphins on circulating concentrations of hyperglycaemic insulin and glucose in dairy cows. *Comparative Biochemistry and Physiology Part A* 127:249–257. [Beta casomorphins infused into gut reduced insulin responses to glucose infusions.]

Koch G, Wiedemann K, Teschemacher H. 1985. Opioid activities of human beta-casomorphins. *Naumyn-Schmiedeberg's Pharmacology* 331:351–354

Lindstrom LH, Lyrenas S, Nyberg F, Terenius L. 1990. Beta-casomorphins in post-partum psychosis. In: F Nyberg and V Brantl (eds), *Beta-casomorphins and related peptides*, pp 157–162. Uppsala: Fyris Tryck.

Meisel H, Fitzgerald RJ. 2000. Opioid peptides encrypted in intact milk protein sequences. *British Journal of Nutrition* 84, Supplement 1: S27–S31.

NHMRC 2003. Infant Feeding Guidelines for Health Workers. Canberra: Australian Health and Medical Research Council.

Norris CS, Darragh A, Booth C, Boland MJ, Hill JP. 2003. Human milks release beta-casomorphin-7 during simulated digestion. *Poster paper presented at the 2003 International Dairy Federation Conference.*

Norris CS, Coker CJ, Boland MJ, Hill JP. 2003. Analysis of the water-soluble fraction of a selection of cheeses for beta-casomorphin, its precursors and its analogues. *Australian Journal of Dairy Technology* 58:201.

Ramabadran K, Bansinath M. 1988. Opioid peptides from milk as a possible cause of sudden infant death syndrome. *Medical Hypotheses* 27(3):181–187.

Shah NP. 2000. Effects of milk-derived bioactives: an overview. *British Journal of Nutrition* 84, Supplement 1: S3–S10.

Sun Z, Zhang Z, Wang X, Cade R, Elmir Z, Fregly M. 2003. Relation of B-casomorphin to apnea in sudden death syndrome. *Peptides* 24(6):937–943

Svedberg J, de Haas J, Leimenstoll G, Paul F, Teschemacher H. 1985. Demonstration of beta-casomorphin immunoreactive materials in *in vitro* digests of bovine milk and in small intestine contents after bovine milk ingestion in adult humans. *Peptides* 6(5):825–830.

Taira T, Hhilakivi LA, Aalto J, Hilakivi I. 1990. Effect of beta casomorphin on neonatal sleep in rats. *Peptides* 11(1):1–4.

Heart Disease

Beaglehole R, Jackson R. 2003. Balancing research for new risk factors and action for the prevention of chronic diseases. *New Zealand Medical Journal* 116(1168).

Biong AS, Veierod MB, Ringstad J, Thelle DS, Pedersen JI. 2006. Intake of milk fat, reflected in adipose tissue fatty acids and risk of myocardial infarction: a case control study. *European Journal of Clinical Nutrition* 60(2):236–244.

Briggs RD, Rubenberg ML, O'Neal RM, Thomas WA, Hartroft WS. 1960. Myocardial infarction in patients treated with Sippy and other high-milk diets *Circulation* 21:538–542.

Chin-Dusting J, Shennan J, Jones E, Williams C, Kingwell B, Dart A. 2006. Effect of dietary supplementation with beta-casein A1 or A2 on markers of disease development in individuals at high risk of cardiovascular disease. *British Journal of Nutrition* 95(1):136–144.

Crawford RA, Boland MJ, Hill JP. 2003. Changes over time in the association between deaths due to ischaemic heart disease and some main food types. *Australian Journal of Dairy Technology* 58:188.

Elwood PC, Pickering JE, Fehily AM, Hughes J, Ness AR. 2004. Milk drinking, ischaemic heart disease and ischaemic stroke 1. Evidence from the Caerphilly cohort. *European Journal of Clinical Nutrition* 58(5):711–717

Hill JP, Crawford RA, Boland MJ. 2002. Milk and consumer health: a review of the evidence for a relationship between the consumption of beta-casein A1 with heart disease and insulin-dependent diabetes mellitus. *Proceedings of the New Zealand Society of Animal Production* 62:111–114.

Hill JP. 2003. The influence of consumption of A1 beta-casein on heart disease and Type 1 diabetes. *New Zealand Medical Journal* 116(1169).

Hill JP, Boland M, Crawford RA, Norris CS. 2003. Changes in milk consumption are not responsible for increase in the incidence of type-1 diabetes or decrease in the incidence of deaths due to ischaemic heart disease. *Australian Journal of Diary Technology* 58:188.

Laugesen M, Elliott R. 2003a. Ischaemic heart disease, Type 1 diabetes, and cow milk A1 beta-casein. *New Zealand Medical Journal* 116(1168).

Laugesen M, Elliott R. 2003b. The influence of consumption of A1 beta-casein on heart disease and Type 1 diabetes – the authors reply. *New Zealand Medical Journal* 116(1170).

Libby P. 2002. Atherosclerosis: the new view. *Scientific American* May, 47–55. [Discusses in non-technical language the link between heart disease and inflammation of the arteries.]

Libby P, Ridker PM, Maseri A. 2002. Inflammation and atherosclerosis. *Circulation* 105(9):1135–1143.

Mann J, Skeaff M. 2003. Editorial – β-casein variants and atherosclerosis – claims are premature. *Atherosclerosis* 170:11–12.

McLachlan CNS. 2003. Setting the record straight: A1 beta-casein, heart disease and diabetes. *New Zealand Medical Journal* 116(1170).

McLachlan CNS. 2001. Beta-casein A1, ischaemic heart disease mortality, and other illnesses. *Medical Hypotheses* 56:262–272.

Owen CG, Whincup PH, Odoki K, Gilg JA, Cook DG. 2002. Infant feeding and blood cholesterol: a study in adolescents and a systematic review. *Pediatrics* 110: 597–608.

Steinerova A, Koretvivka M, Racek J, Rajdl D, Trefil L, Stozicky F, Rokyta Z. 2004. Letter to the Editor: Significant increase in antibodies against oxidized LDL particles (IgoxLDL) in three-month old infants who received milk formulae. *Atherosclerosis* 173(1):147–148.

Steinerova A, Racek J, Stozicky F, Tatzber F. 1999. Autoantibodies against LDL in the first phase of life. *Clinical Chemistry and Laboratory Medicine* 37(9):913–917.

Steinerova A, Stozicky F, Racek J, Tatzber F, Zima T, Setina R. 2001. Antibodies against LDL in infants. *Clinical Chemistry* 47(6):1137–1138. [Showed a statistically strong ($p< 0.001$) relationship between LDL antibodies and whether breast-fed or formula fed.]

Tailford KA, Berry CL, Thomas AC and Campbell JH. 2003. A casein variant in cow's milk is atherogenic. *Atherosclerosis* 170:13–19.

Torreilles J, Guerin MC. 1995. Casein-derived peptides promote peroxidase-dependent oxidation of human blood low-density lipoproteins. *Comptes Rendus Seances de la Société Biologie Fil* 189:933–942. [In French).

Venn BJ, Skeaff CM, Brown R, Mann JI, Green TJ. 2006. A comparison of the effects of A1 and A2 beta-casein protein variants on blood cholesterol concentrations in New Zealand adults. *Atherosclerosis* 188:175–178.

Diabetes

Beales PE, Elliott RB, Flohé S, Hill JP, Kolb H, Pozzilli P, Wang GS, Wasmuth H, Scott FW. 2002. A multi-centre, blinded international trial of the effect of A1 and A2 beta casein variants on diabetes incidence in two rodent models of spontaneous Type 1 diabetes. *Diabetologia* 45:1240–1246.

Birgisdottir BE, Hill JP, Thorsson AV, Thorsdottir I. 2006. Lower consumption of cow milk protein A1 beta-casein at 2 years of age, rather than among 11–14-year-old adolescents, may explain the lower incidence of type 1 diabetes in Iceland than in Scandinavia. *Annals of Nutrition and Metabolism* 50(3):177–183.

Birgisdottir BE, Hill JP, Harris DP, Thorsdottir I. 2002. Variation in consumption of cow milk proteins and lower incidence of Type 1 diabetes in Iceland vs the other 4 Nordic countries. *Diabetes, Nutrition and Metabolism* 15(4):240–245.

Elliott R, Wasmuth H, Bibby N, Hill J. 1997. The role of beta-casein variants in the induction of insulin-dependent diabetes in the non-obese diabetic mouse and humans. In: *Milk Protein Polymorphism* Special Issue 9702:445–453 Brussels: International Dairy Federation.

Elliott RB. 2006. Diabetes – a man-made disease. *Medical Hypotheses* 67:388–391. [Discusses glycation products including glycated BCM7 as an explanation for the increase in diabetes.]

Elliott RB, Martin JM. 1984. Dietary protein: a trigger of insulin-dependent diabetes in the BB rat? *Diabetologia* 26:297–299.

Elliott RB, Harris DP, Hill JP, Bibby NJ, Wasmuth HE. 1999. Type 1 (insulin dependent) diabetes mellitus and cow milk: casein variant consumption. *Diabetologia* 42:292–296.

Hill JP, Crawford RA, Boland MJ. 2002. Milk and consumer health: a review of the evidence for a relationship between the consumption of beta-casein A1 with heart disease and insulin-dependent diabetes mellitus. *Proceedings of the New Zealand Society of Animal Production* 62:111–114.

Hill JP. 2003. The influence of consumption of A1 beta-casein on heart disease and Type 1 diabetes. *New Zealand Medical Journal* 116(1169).

Hill JP, Boland M, Crawford RA, Norris CS. 2003. Changes in milk consumption are not responsible for increase in the incidence of type-1 diabetes or decrease in the incidence of deaths due to ischaemic heart disease. *Australian Journal of Diary Technology* 58:188.

Hoppe C, Molgaard C, Vaag A, Barkholt V, Michaelsen KF. 2005. High intakes of milk, but not meat, increase s-insulin and insulin resistance in 8-year-old boys. *European Journal of Clinical Nutrition* 59:393–398.

Laugesen M, Elliott R. 2003a. Ischaemic heart disease, Type 1 diabetes, and cow milk A1 beta-casein. *New Zealand Medical Journal* 116(1168).

Laugesen M, Elliott R. 2003b. The influence of consumption of A1 beta-casein on heart disease and Type 1 diabetes – the authors reply. *New Zealand Medical Journal* 1169(1170).

Norris JM, Barriga K, Klingensmith G, Hoffman M, Eisenbarth GS, Erlich HA, Rewers M. 2003. Timing of initial cereal exposure in infancy and risk of islet autoimmunity. *Journal of the American Medical Association*. 290(13):1713–1720.

Onkamo P, Vaananen S, Karvonem M, Tuomelihto J. 1999. Worldwide increase in incidence of Type 1 diabetes – the analysis of the data on published incidence trends. *Diabetologia* 42:1395–1403.

Padberg S, Schumm-Draeger PM, Petzoldt R, Becker F, Federlin K. 1999. The significance of A1 and A2 antibodies against beta-casein in Type 1 diabetes mellitus. *Deutsch Medizinische Wochenschrift* 124(50):1518-21 [Found very strong evidence ($p< 0.001$) of antibodies against A1 beta-casein in Type 1 diabetics.]

Pozzilli P, Signore A, Williams AJ, Beales PE. 1993. NOD mouse colonies around the world – recent facts and figures. *Immunology Today* 14:193–196.

Pozzilli P. 2004. Product derived from milk substantially free of beta casein from non-human mammals and relative use. United States Patent 6,750,203. PCT Pub No WO97/24371.

Pozzilli P. 1999. Beta-casein in cow's milk: a major antigenic determinant for Type 1 diabetes? *Journal of Endocrinological Investigation* 22:562–567.

Scott FW, Kolb H. 2003. A1 beta-casein milk and Type 1 diabetes: causal relationship probed in animal models. *New Zealand Medical Journal* 116(1170).

Thorsdottir I, Birgisdottir BE, Johannsdottir IM, Harris DP, Hill J, Steingrimsdottir L, Thorsson AV. 2002. Different beta-casein fractions in Iceland vs Scandinavian cow's milk may influence diabetogenicity of cow's milk in infancy and explain the low incidence of insulin-dependent diabetes mellitus (IDDM) in Iceland. *Pediatrics* 106:719–724.

Virtanen S, Laara E, Hypponen E, Reijonen, H, Rasanen L, Aro A, Knip M, Ilonen J, Akerblom, HK. 2000. Cow's milk consumption, HLA-DQB1 genotype, and Type 1 diabetes: a nested case-control study of siblings of children with diabetes. *Diabetes* 40:912–917. [Subsequently there was an erratum printed in the September 2000 issue of *Diabetes*]

Autism and Schizophrenia

Cade R, Privette M, Fregly M, Rowland N, Sun Z, Zele V, Wagemaker H, Edelstein C. 2000. Autism and schizophrenia: intestinal disorders. *Nutritional Neuroscience* 3:57–72.

Christison GW, Ivany K. 2006. Elimination diets in autism spectrum disorders: any wheat amongst the chaff. *Journal of Developmental & Behavioral Pediatrics.* 27(2Suppl):S162–171.

Dohan FC. 1988. Genetic hypothesis of idiopathic schizophrenia: its exorphin connection. *Schizophrenia Bulletin* 14(4):489–494. [Dohan was the first person to link schizophrenia with nutrition. His first report is dated 1966.]

Elder JH, Shankar M, Shuster J, Theriaque D, Burns S, Sherrill L. 2006. The gluten-free casein-free diet in autism: results of a preliminary double blind clinical trial. *Journal of Autism and Developmental Disorders* 36(3):413–420.

Knivsberg A-M, Reichelt KL, Hoien T, Nodland M. 2002. A randomized, controlled study of dietary intervention in autistic syndromes. *Nutritional Neuroscience* 5:251–261.

Knivsberg AM, Reichelt KL, Nodland M. 2001. Reports on dietary intervention in autistic disorders. *Nutritional Neuroscience* 4:23–27.

Knivsberg A-M, Reichelt KL, Nodland M, Hoien T. 1995. Autistic syndromes and diet: a follow-up study. *Scandinavian Journal of Education Research* 39:223–236.

New Zealand Dairy Research Institute. 2001. Milk containing beta-casein with proline at position 67 does not aggravate neurological disorders. International Patent Number WO 02/19832 A1. (PCT/NZ01/00186). [This patent application was subsequently abandoned.]

Panksepp J. 1979. A neurochemical theory of autism. *Trends in Neuroscience* 2:174–177.

Reichelt KL, Ekrem J, Scott H. 1990. Gluten, milk proteins, and autism: dietary intervention effects on behaviour and peptide secretion. *Journal of Applied Nutrition* 42:1–11.

Reichelt KL, Knivsberg A-M. 2003. Can the pathophysiology of autism be explained by the nature of the discovered urine peptides? *Nutritional Neuroscience* 6:19–28.

Reichelt KL, Skjeldal O. 2006. IgA antibodies and Rett syndrome. *Autism* 10(2):189–197.

Reichelt WH, Stensrud EJ, MB, Reichelt KL. 1998. Peptide excretion in celiac disease. *Journal of Pediatric Gastroenterology and Nutrition* 26:305–309.

Shattock P, Kennedy A, Rowell F, Berney T. 1990. Role of neuropeptides in autism and their relationships with classical transmitters. *Brain Dysfunction* 3:328–346.

Sponheim E, Myhre AM, Reichelt KL, Aalen OO. 2006. Urine peptide patterns in children with milder types of autism. *Tidsskrift for den Norske Laegeforening* 126(11):1475–1477. [English language Abstract with the main paper in Norwegian.]

Sun Z, Cade JR. 1999. A peptide found in schizophrenia and autism causes behavioural changes in rats. *Autism* 3(1)85–95. [Reports trial evidence for injected BCM7 causing strong behavioural changes in rats.]

Sun Z, Cade JR, Fregly MJ, Privette RM. 1999. Beta casomorphin induces Fos-like immunoreactivity in discrete brain regions relevant to schizophrenia and autism. *Autism* 3(1):67–83 [Presents evidence that BCM7 can cross the blood/brain barrier, activate opioid receptors and affect brain regions similar to those affected by schizophrenia and autism]

Sun Z, Cade JR. 2003. Findings in normal rats following administration of gliadorphin-7 (GD-7). *Peptides* 24(2):321–323. [Found that gliadorphin (GD-7) affects only three regions of the brains, cf. 45 regions for BCM7. Also that 'GD-7 gains access to brain cells by diffusion through circumventricular organs while BCM-7 passes the BBB [blood/brain barrier] by carrier facilitation.' GD-7 caused no behavioural change whereas BCM7 'causes bizarre behavior'.]

Wei J, Hemmings GP. 2005. Gene, gut and schizophrenia: the meeting point for the gene-environment interaction in developing schizophrenia. *Medical Hypotheses* 64(3):547–552.

Allergies, Intolerance and Auto-immune Conditions

Agranoff BW, Goldberg D. 1974. Diet and the geographical distribution of multiple sclerosis. *Lancet* 2(7888):1061–1066.

Bushara KO. 2005. Neurologic presentation of coeliac disease. *Gastroenterology* 128(4 Pt2): S92–97.

Chen H, Zhang SM, Hernan MA, Willett WC, Ascherio A. 2002. Diet and Parkinson's disease: a potential role of dairy products in men. *Annals of Neurology* 53:793–801.

Chen H, O'Reilly E, McCullough ML, Rodriguez C, Schwarzschild MA, Calle EE, Thun MJ, Ascherio A. 2007. Consumption of dairy products and risk of Parkinson's disease. *American Journal of Epidemiology* 165(9):998–1006.

Dorman JS, Steenkiste AR, Burke JP, Songini M. 2003. Type 1 diabetes and multiple sclerosis: together at last. *Diabetes Care* 26:3192–3193.

Eaton WW, Mortensen PB, Agerbo E, Byrne M, Mors O, Ewald H. 2004. Coeliac disease and schizophrenia: population based case control study with linkage of Danish national registers. *British Medical Journal* 328:438–439.

Gearry RB, Richardson A, Frampton CM, Collett JA, Burt MJ, Chapman BA, Barclay ML. 2006. High incidence of Crohn's disease in Canterbury, New Zealand: results of an epidemiologic study. *Inflammatory Bowel Disease* 12(10):936–943.

Geissler A, Andus T, Roth M, Kullmann F, Caesar I, Held P, Gross V, Fuerbach S, Scholmerich J. 1995. Focal white-matter lesions in brains of patients with inflammatory bowel disease. *Lancet* 345(8954):897–898.

Lai BCL, Tsui JKC. 2001. Epidemiology of Parkinson's disease. *British Columbia Medical Journal* 43(3):133–137.

Lauer K. 1994. The risk of multiple sclerosis in the USA in relation to sociogeographic features: a factor analytic study. *Journal of Clinical Epidemiology* 47:43–48.

Malekzadeh R, Sachdev A, Fahid A. 2005. Coeliac disease in developing countries: Middle east, India, and North Africa. *Best Practice Research in Clinical Gastroenterology* 19(3):351–358.

Malosse D. 1992. Correlation between milk and dairy product consumption and multiple sclerosis prevalence: a worldwide study. *Neuroepidemiology* 1194(6):304–312.

Marrosu MG, Cocco E, Lai M, Spinicci G, Pischedda MP, Contu P. 2002. Patients with multiple sclerosis and risk of Type 1 diabetes mellitus in Sardinia: a cohort study. *Lancet* 359(9316):1461–1465.

Marrosu MG, Lampis R, Costa G, Zavattari P, Contu D, Fadda E, Cocco E, Cucca F. 2004. The co-inheritance of Type 1 diabetes and multiple sclerosis in Sardinia cannot be explained by genotype variation in the HLA region alone. *Human Molecular Genetics* 13(23):2919–2924.

Monetini L, Cavallo MG, Manfrini S, Stefanini L, Picarelli A, Di Tola M, Petrone A, Bianchi M, La Presa M, Di Giulio C, Baroni MG, Thorpe R, Walter BK, Pozzilli P. 2002. Antibodies to bovine beta-casein and other autoimmune diseases. *Hormonal and Metabolic Research* 34(8):455–459.

Park M, Ross GW, Petrovich H, White LR, Masaki KH, Nelson MD, Tanner CM, Curb JD, Planchette PL, Abbott RD. 2005. Consumption of milk and calcium in midlife and the future risk of Parkinson's disease. *Neurology* 64:1051–1056.

Reichelt K-L, Jensen D. 2004. IgA antibodies against gliadin and gluten in multiple sclerosis. *Acta Neurologica Scandinavica* 110(4):239–241. [Also measured significantly higher antibodies to casein in persons suffering from MS.]

Ross GW, Abbott RD, Petrovitch H, Morens DM, Grandinetti A, Tung KH, Tanner CM, Masaki KH, Blanchette PL, Curb JD, Popper JS, White LR. 2000. Association of coffee and caffeine intake with the risk of Parkinson's disease. *Journal of the American Medical Association* 283(20):2674–2679.

Shabo Y, Barzel R, Margoulis M, Yagil R. 2005. Camel milk for food allergies in children. *Israel Medical Association Journal* 7(12):796–798.

Smith WB, Thompson D, Kummerow M, Quinn P, Gold MS. 2004. A2 milk is allergenic. *Medical Journal of Australia* 181(10):574.

Sun Z, Zhang Z, Wang X, Cade R, Elmir Z, Fregly M. 2003. Relation of beta-casomorphin to apnea in sudden infant death syndrome. *Peptides* 24(6):937–943.

Ventura A, Magazzu G, Greco L. 1999. Duration of exposure to gluten and risk for autoimmune disorders inpatients with celiac disease. SIGEP Study Group for Autoimmune Disorders in Celiac disease. *Gastroenterology* 117(2):297–303. [Showed that coeliac sufferers and Crohn's disease sufferers had higher levels of other auto-immune diseases than age-matched controls.]

Winer S, Astsaturov I, Cheung R, Gunaratnam L, Kubiak V, Cortez MA, Moscarello M, O'Connor PW, McKerlie C, Becker DJ, Dosch HM. 2001. Type 1 diabetes and multiple sclerosis patients target islet plus central nervous system autoantigens; nonimmunized non obese diabetic mice develop autoimmune encephalitis. *Journal of Immunology* 166(4):2831–2841.

Zoghbi S, Trompette A, Claustre J, El Homsi M, Garzon J, Jourdain G, Scoazec J, Plaisancie P. 2006. B-casomorphin-7 regulates the secretion and expression of gastrointestinal mucins through a mu-opioid pathway. *American Journal of Physiology. Gastrointestinal and Liver Physiology* 290:G1105–G1113.

Cattle Genetics

Bradley DG, Loftus RT, Cunningham P, MacHugh DE. 1998. Genetics and domestic cattle origins. *Evolutionary Anthropology,* 6:79–86.

Formaggioni P, Dummer A, Malacarne M, Mariani P. 1999. Milk protein polymorphism: detection and diffusion of the genetic variants in *Bos* genus. *Vol X1X Universiti degli Studi de Parma, Annalli della Facolta di Medicina Veterinaria.*

Ng-Kwai-Hang KF, Grosclaude F. 2002. Genetic polymorphism of milk proteins. In: PF Fox and McSweeney PLH (eds), *Advanced Dairy Chemistry*, 737–814, Kluwer Academic/Plenum Publishers, New York.

Woodford, KB. 2004. A2 milk and farmer decisions. *Primary Industry Management* 7(3):26–27.

Morris CA, Hickey SM, Cullen NG, Prosser CG, Anderson RM, Tate ML. 2005. Associations between beta-casein genotype and milk yield and composition in grazing dairy cows. *New Zealand Journal of Agricultural Research* 48:441–450.

Industry, Marketing and Overview

Australian Broadcasting Corporation. 2003. White Mischief. Available at http://www.abc.net.au/4corners/content/2003/transcripts/s820943.htm

Clarke AJ, Allison AJ. 2006. Further research for consideration in 'the A2 milk case'. *European Journal of Clinical Nutrition* 60(7):921–924.

Cone, DH. 2003. Secret memo reveals Fonterra's alarm. *National Business Review.* Available at www.sharechat.co.nz/features/nbr/article.php/569e538.

Harvard School of Public Health. 2006. Calcium and milk. Available at www.hsph.harvard.edu/nutritionsources/calcium.html

MacNeill I. 2003. Marketing of dairy messages. *Australian Journal of Dairy Technology* 58(2):126–128.

Swinburn B. 2004. Beta casein A1 and A2 in milk and human health. Report to New Zealand Food Safety Authority. Available at www.nzsfa.govt.nz [NB. There is both a separate Lay Summary and a considerably more lengthy main report.]

Truswell AS. 2005. The A2 milk case: a critical review. *European Journal of Clinical Nutrition* 59:623–631.

Truswell AS. 2006. Reply: the A2 milk case. *European Journal of Clinical Nutrition* 60(7):924–925.

Woodford KB. 2004(a). The A2 milk debate: searching for the evidence. *Primary Industry Management* 7(4):29–33. Also available at: www.lincoln.ac.nz/story_images/837_a2milk_s3292.pdf

Woodford KB. 2004(b) A2 milk. Guest editorial in *Bioscience News*, 24 March 2004. Originally available at www.bioscnews.com Currently available at: www.lincoln.ac.nz/story_images/838_a2milk_s3293.pdf

Woodford KB. 2004(c). A2 milk debate unlikely to go away. *Food New Zealand.* April 2004: 12.

Woodford KB. 2006. A critique of Truswell's A2 milk review. *European Journal of Clinical Nutrition.* 60(3):437–439.

APPENDIX ONE

Some principles of medical investigation

The basis of the scientific method

Medical science is based on the scientific method. A key element of the scientific method is that science should be evidence-based and objective. Accordingly, trials are based on testing hypotheses, which themselves are based on prior knowledge, logical reasoning and observations.

Trials must be set up so that hypotheses have the potential to be proven either true or false. However, trial results often lead not so much to proving something true or false in any absolute sense, but to a more refined and sophisticated hypothesis that can be further tested. This is consistent with the notion that science moves forward by incremental steps. Scientists are expected to archive and share all data, plus methodology, so that others can scrutinise their work.

Randomised trials

Randomised trials are the most persuasive form of investigation for demonstrating causality between treatment and effect. They involve dividing trial participants randomly into at least two groups, one of which is subjected to the 'treatment' and the other group is a 'control' group whose members are given placebos. Wherever possible, participants in a trial are kept unaware ('blind') as to whether they are receiving the treatment or the control. It is also desirable that the investigators taking the measurements are also unaware ('blind') as to who is receiving the treatment and who is receiving the placebo until all analyses have been completed. This is to eliminate investigator bias, which can be either subconscious or conscious. Subconscious bias is particularly important when measuring something subjective (for example, 'wellness').

Crossover trials are a special form of randomised trial where some participants initially receive the real treatment and others receive the control (placebo), and then the groups swap over after a period of, for example, six weeks.

Randomised trials work well where the treatment is short-term and where the treatment is a drug, so that it is easy to disguise which people are receiving the drug and which are getting the placebo. However, for long-term investigations, such as of the auto-immune conditions which can have latency periods of 30 years or more, random trials are difficult and usually impossible to execute. Also, for many treatments, such as comparing smoking with non-smoking, or milk consumption with non-milk consumption, it can be impossible to disguise who is receiving which treatment.

Clinical trials

Clinical trials are a type of randomised trial used in drug testing and some other forms of clinical intervention. Typically there are three phases. Phase 1 involves testing the treatment on healthy volunteers. The focus is on safety of the treatment, not whether it is effective. This phase 1 trial will typically have been preceded by pre-clinical trials on animals. Phase 2 involves testing the effects of the drug on a moderate number of people (possibly several hundred). Phase 3 involves large-scale randomised trials. All trials involving humans require ethical approval from an appropriate regulatory body. The total process from pre-clinical testing in animals to completion of phase 3 trials takes typically 10 years or more.

Between-country epidemiological studies

These are also called ecological studies. They are based on statistical analyses of between-country disease-incidence relationships and various dietary and lifestyle factors in those countries. These studies, if properly conducted, can be very powerful in providing evidence but by themselves are usually regarded as being insufficient to prove cause. A key starting point is to make sure that the criteria used for measuring incidence of the disease in question are consistent between countries. For diseases such as Type 1 diabetes this is not a problem but for diseases such as multiple sclerosis and Parkinson's disease it can be problematic.

The second issue is that it is possible for confounding to occur because of the multiplicity of lifestyle differences between countries. Well-conducted studies therefore test for all conceivable factors, not just the suspected factor. Also, well-conducted studies typically try to compare countries that have similar overall levels of development, and similar standards of healthcare. Epidemiologists make use of statistical procedures to test whether the relationships that they find are likely to be real effects or just due to random variation.

Cohort studies

Cohort studies are another form of epidemiology. Typically they are long-term studies of large groups of people (typically many thousands) for up to 30 years or even more. The participants are free to choose their own lifestyles and diets, but they record what they eat, drink and do. Epidemiologists then track the various disease conditions that they develop, and undertake statistical tests to identify which diseases are associated with which lifestyle factors. Some of the most informative studies have been of health professionals, who tend to be easier than other people to keep track of over a long period.

One of the problems with cohort studies is that particular lifestyle factors tend to be associated with each other. For example, health-conscious people tend to not smoke and tend to exercise, to take vitamin tablets and to drink fat-reduced milk. Teasing out causation can therefore be very difficult.

Case control

Case-control studies involve a group of people who have a disease, and comparing these people with a group of apparently similar people (in terms of age and socioeconomic status) who do not have the disease. The comparison might involve getting the individuals from both the case and control groups to describe their lifestyles many years ago to see whether there is indeed something that sets the sufferers apart from the healthy participants. The problem here is ensuring accurate recall. Another approach is to take biochemical measurements on the two different groups to see, for example, whether they show antibody differences relating to particular proteins.

Case histories and observations

This form of evidence is the least scientific because it lacks controls and relies on accuracy of recall. Nevertheless, in practice many doctors rely on case histories, including their own clinical experiences. Case histories and observations should always include as much detail as possible relating to what, when, how, and under what conditions. Well-documented case histories and observations, despite their limitations, are published in many peer-reviewed journals. Scientists who denigrate case histories and observations sometimes refer to them as 'anecdotes' which essentially means 'stories'. The term 'anecdote' is best reserved for situations where good documentation on what, when, how, and under what conditions is not provided. Case histories tend to be much more valuable if the measures are explicit (such as laboratory measurement of blood parameters, or diarrhoea) rather than subjective judgements (such as 'wellness') which can be notoriously unreliable.

Animal trials

Given the difficulties in conducting trials in humans, it is common to use animals as surrogates. These trials have to be approved by animal welfare regulatory authorities. The problem with using animals is that biochemical processes can be different between animals and humans. However, there is also a great deal that is common between humans and animals. A trial in animals can therefore never by itself prove what will happen in humans but it can provide important indications and insights. Animal trials are often undertaken using dose rates that are much higher than would be experienced in normal human diets in an attempt to get a quick effect.

In vitro laboratory studies

In vitro means 'in the test tube' (as opposed to *in vivo*, which means 'in the living organism'). These studies typically involve biochemically testing particular tissues or substances, taken from humans and animals. *In vitro* experiments include measuring digestion products when foods are exposed to specific digestive enzymes. Such studies are particularly valuable for investigating the underlying science and biochemical mechanisms, but some caution has to be exercised in interpreting the results as living and artificial situations are not always quite the same.

Statistical significance

Statistics is an important field that causes huge confusion, not only amongst lay people but also amongst many scientists themselves. Statistical procedures are used to test the reliability of data analysed from a sample of people (the trial participants) and therefore whether the conclusions drawn can be said to apply to the broader population as well.

The reason this is such an important issue is that different people react differently to the same drug or chemical or food. Hence, we have to investigate whether any measured difference is likely to have been caused by chance selection of particular trial participants with particular susceptabilities.

When statisticians say that a result is significant at $p< 0.05$ (or alternatively worded, at the 5% level) they are saying that if there were no real difference in the broad population between the effects of treatment and control, then we should expect to get a 'fluke result' like this, through chance selection of particular trial participants, less than one time in 20. And if a result is significant at $p< 0.01$, then if there is no real difference between treatment and control, we would only expect to get an experimental result as strong as this in less than one in one hundred trials.

The classic statistics that are used in medical science place the major emphasis on trying to avoid a situation where we think we have found a real difference when we have not. This is called a Type 1 error. This error occurs when we say that the effects of the trial are 'significant', implying that a difference exists in the overall population, when in fact (but unknown to the investigator) the difference is caused by chance and hence unlikely to be repeatable in further trials.

Type 2 errors are the reverse of this. They occur when it is said that no significant differences were obtained but in fact there are (unknown to the investigators) real differences between the treatment and control which the trial, through chance selection of participants, has either failed to identify at all, or has identified but failed to identify as being significant.

There is always a trade off in statistical analyses between Type 1 and Type 2 errors. In trying to reduce the chance of a Type 1 error to no more than one in 20 we inevitably increase the likelihood of making Type 2 errors.

Accordingly, when measured differences are said to be non-significant that does not mean that they are not real. It simply means that the experiment had insufficient power to identify with confidence that the measured differences were indeed real. If these differences look potentially important then the message has to be that another trial needs to be done with more power. One way to increase the power of a trial is to get a larger number of participants.

There are, of course, other factors apart from Type 2 errors that can lead to the failure to identify real differences. If a trial is poorly designed, so that the wrong measurements are taken, or measuring equipment is incorrectly calibrated, then the data are faulty and no statistical technique can rectify the problem (hence the saying 'garbage in, garbage out'). Also, if a trial is designed, for whatever reason, with a low level of discriminatory power, then we can be confident in advance that the results will be non-significant.

Correlation and causation

One of the accepted tenets of statistics is that just because two variables are correlated does not mean that there is causation involved. There are two reasons for this. The first is that the correlation might be caused by chance or random 'noise' in the data. Accordingly, when an apparent correlation between variables is found, tests need to be done to determine the significance of the correlation.

Even if a relationship is found to be significant and hence unlikely to be a chance relationship, there is a need to be very careful in saying that A is caused by B. Instead it may be that B is caused by A, or that both A and B are caused by a third factor, C.

Perhaps the key message, however, is that although significant correlations do not prove causation, these significant correlations should never be dismissed as unimportant. The fact that they are statistically significant means that it is unlikely that such results would arise by chance.

Peer review

Peer review is the process whereby scientific work is reviewed, typically by scientists who are independent of those undertaking the work, prior to publication. Peer reviewers are typically chosen by the journal editors and their anonymity is usually preserved from the authors.

The peer-review process is designed to stop scientists drawing conclusions from their work that are not supported by the data. Reviewers typically look first at the logic of the research hypothesis. They will then review the research protocol and methods in relation to their appropriateness for investigating the hypothesis. They will then look at the results and whether the statistical methods were appropriate. It is not normal for peer reviewers to look at the original data themselves, or to check for fraud or non-disclosure.

Most commonly, a journal will invite two scientists to conduct a review independently of each other, and to provide a report. The editor will then make a judgement to accept the paper, to reject it, or to ask for modification.

Peer review is a very important part of science but it can also be a 'lottery'. Reviewers are themselves very busy people, and conducting peer reviews tends to be considered a chore. It undoubtedly prevents a lot of rubbish from being published, but there is still a great deal of flawed science that gets through. History also shows that sometimes it is the most important findings, that contradict accepted wisdom, that get ensnared in the review process.

Almost all scientists support the principle of peer review. But there is a lot of debate amongst scientists as to how it might be done better.

The big picture

There is no one way to undertake medical research. Some issues can be investigated using randomised trials, and where this is the case then it is the way that the science should be conducted. But if science were to accept only results that came out of randomised trials, then science would progress very slowly.

In real life, science and medicine progress by using a combination of approaches. That includes ecological epidemiology, cohort investigations, case-control studies, case histories, animal trials and *in-vitro* studies. In finding answers to the disease problems that afflict humankind we need to use every tool at our disposal.

APPENDIX TWO

October 2000 briefing paper by Dr Jeremy Hill, NZDRI, for NZ Dairy Board CEO Warren Larsen

Paragraph layout, spelling and grammar have been retained as in the original memo.

Briefing Paper on A2 Corporation
Summary

In my opinion:

The scientific validity of A2 Corporations claims that A1 milk is strongly correlated with heart disease is weak.

The claim that A2 Corporation can get around the NZDB patent position is very doubtful.

The science that there is an effect of A1 or A2 milks on the development of diseases or disorders is still unproven, but is the subject of ongoing NZDB funded work.

No health claims on A1 or A2 milk could be made at this time and used to aid marketing of these milks.

There is growing evidence, but yet unproven that peptides released from milk may be related to occurrence of some mental disorders.

If the media (or A2 Corporation) were ever able to assemble the information shown in this paper they could put an alarmist spin on the whole area of milk consumption or alternatively leap to conclusions about A1 vs A2 effects before a case is proven either way.

Taken in totality the contents of this briefing paper could form the basis of an argument for the production of A2 milks and milk products for at risk individuals. However, who may be at risk is still unclear and a diagnostic or diagnostics is a priority. The presence of beta-casomorphin-7 in urine holds some hope in this respect.

The NZ dairy industry has all of the capabilities needed to produce A1 or A2 type milks without the need for outside assistance.

A2 milks could be marketed and distributed through health retail outlets (chemist/health food shops) and in so doing keep their distribution and marketing away from normal milk.

Does A2 really have any significant scientific findings?

A2 claim that they have intellectual property relating to a strong link between the consumption of A1 milk and heart disease. This is based as far as we are aware on epidemiology only.

NZDRI even dispute the epidemiology and cannot find the strong relationship that A2 propose.

A2 have tried to publish this work, but have not been able to. This suggests that the referees of the journals to which they sent the work are not convinced about the science.

They have produced statements from so-called referees who praise the work. I would suggest that these referees do not understand the inadequacy of the data that has been used to draw conclusions.

The inadequacy of the data on the actual amount of A1 variant consumed in a particular country makes the scientific claims A2 Corporation very questionable.

A2 Corp. claim that they have evidence that casein is getting into the blood stream and that this is the cause of the problem. This is common knowledge and probably has nothing to do with their claims.

A2 Corp. have proposed a variety of possible mechanisms to explain their observations. None of these appears to be likely and often demonstrate a poor understanding of both dairy chemistry and physiology by A2 Corp.

Can A2 Corporation get around the NZDB Patent?

A2 Corp. claim that the NZDB patent position does not cover the genotyping of animals or the selection of animals for segregation.

The NZDB patent specifically covers genotyping (typing from DNA) and phenotyping (typing from milk).

The NZDB patent is also very comprehensive with respect to the selection of animals and we have discussed this many times with Doug Calhoun from A J Park to make sure that we have not left any loopholes. There are no loopholes and we are sure that the patent could be defended in court.

The NZDB patent position predates that of A2 Corporation.

The NZDB patent covers the class of A1 type milks (A1, B and C etc) and A2 type milks (A2 and A3 etc).

The A2 Corp. patent covers only A1 type milk and claims that other milk particularly A2 should be fine. This we think is because A2 Corp. did not and do not understand the basis of how A1 and A2 milks might have a different biological activity.

It could be claimed that A2 Corp. obtained from the NZDRI/Bob Elliott some information (Icelandic milk composition) and the concept of looking at the relationship between variant milk consumptions and diseases before this became publicly available. Permission was not given by the NZDB and NZDRI and Bob Elliott claims that he also did not give permission.

Does the NZDB have any significant scientific findings?

The background to this whole area originates from a phone conversation between Bob Elliott and myself in 1993. Bob had phoned the NZDRI and asked to speak with someone who knew something about cows. Bob told me that he thought that casein might be triggering diabetes and asked me if all cows were the same. Upon finding that diabetes was an auto-immune disease and knowing that beta-casein in milk released an immune reactive peptide and that there was a difference in the sequence of this peptide in beta-casein A1 and A2, I suggested to Bob that there might be a difference in the effect of these types of casein on the development of diabetes, although at the time I thought this to be an extremely long shot.

Under an NZDB funded project NZDRI supplied A1 and A2 caseins for Elliott to feed to diabetes prone mice.

Only those mice fed A1 developed diabetes.

This result formed the basis of the joint NZDB/Child Health Research Foundation (CHRF) patent.

The results have also been broadly published.

Soon after this, work by a German group showed that the bioactive peptide beta-casomorphin-7 (BCM-7) could only be released from A1 type variants (A1, B and C etc) and not A2 type variants (A2 and A3 etc).

This makes perfect mechanistic sense given the differences between A1 and A2 as the proline at position 67 in the A2 variant makes this bond resistant to hydrolysis by digestive enzymes unlike the histidine at this position in the A1 variant.

Under NZDB funding we hired a German researcher to work with Bob Elliott to look at the effect of BCM-7 on the activity of immune cells isolated from humans.
BCM-7 inhibited the activity of immune cells from pre-diabetics and actually activated immune cells from normal humans.

This work formed the basis of a second NZDB/CHRF patent on a potential diagnostic for diabetes and also a recent patent application by the NZDB on potential positive effects of A1 milk.

The work was broadly published.

It was also clear that Iceland stood out as an anomaly in that it had one of the highest per capita consumptions of milk yet a moderate level of diabetes.

NZDRI established collaboration with Icelandic researchers to study the composition of Iceland milk under NZDB funding.
Unlike the milk from most other countries which contains approximately equal amounts of the A1 and A2 types of variants, Icelandic milk was approximately 75% A2 and only 25% A1.

An NZDB funded study was performed to look at the relationship between the consumption of A1 type milks and diabetes in a number of countries where we had some confidence of:

1. The diabetes incidence in those countries.
2. The amount of A1 and other beta-casein variants in the milk supply.
3. A limited (<5%) amount of milk was imported from other countries.

A strong relationship between the consumption of A1 milk and diabetes was observed, which became even stronger for the relationship between A1+B milk and diabetes. That is the per capita consumption of two most common variants which can release BCM-7 is strongly correlated with diabetes. This work was published in the international journal Diabetologia.

However, a number of assumptions were made (as is always the case) in constructing the relationship, and as with all epidemiology, the correlation does not prove a cause and effect relationship.

Under NZDB funding NZDRI has since worked with the Icelandic group to investigate in more detail the composition of Nordic milks and the relationship to diabetes in those countries. In general the earlier relationship (*Diabetologia* paper) appears to hold true. This work has been accepted for publication in the international journal *Pediatrics.*

To further investigate if Bob Elliott's feeding trial results could be duplicated a large NZDB funded multi-laboratory multi-national trial was performed – the Food and Diabetes (FAD) Trial. In this trial coded diets supplied from the NZDRI were fed to diabetes prone rats and mice in Auckland (Elliott), Canada and the UK. Groups in Italy, Germany, and the US also collaborated in the trial.

The effects observed by Elliott were not consistently repeated in the FAD Trial and in fact were shown in only one case, in rats in the Canadian laboratory.

An important result observed in the trial was that cereal-based diets produced much higher levels of diabetes than the milk based diets in all laboratories.

Another important result from the trial was that a hypoallergenic infant formula (Pregestimil) also produced high levels of diabetes.

NZDRI has since shown that Pregestimil contains a high amount of BCM-7. This result is not known outside the NZ dairy industry and forms the basis of a confidential NZDRI Report.

Note that gluten containing cereals can also release a BCM-7-like peptide.

The results from the FAD Trial were presented at two large international diabetes conferences and are currently being produced as a paper for publication in the international literature.
Work performed with rats by US researchers has shown that BCM-7 binds to brain cells via morphine receptor sites on brain cells.

The US group found that when BCM-7 was injected into the rats they exhibited marked behaviour changes akin to schizophrenia. The effect of BCM-7 could be blocked by the drug Naloxone which prevents the BCM-7 from binding to the morphine receptor sites.

It is significant that the effect of A1 on the development of diabetes in Elliott's mouse colony was also blocked by giving the mice Naloxone in their drinking water. This result has been published.

NZDRI has shown that there is a relationship between the consumption of A1 and deaths due to mental disorders. This is only based on epidemiology, but might be possible if BCM-7 effects brain function as suggested by the US work with rats. The relationship forms the basis of a patent application by NZDB (covers mental disorders including autism and schizophrenia).

There has been circumstantial evidence that the removal of milk and gluten containing cereals from the diet can reduce or alleviate the symptoms of autism in some children.

A recent patent by a US company has shown that in two thirds of autistic children examined, BCM-7 and the equivalent peptides from gluten could be found in their urine but not in the urine from normal individuals.

The patent could form the basis of a diagnostic for the targeting of people who are at risk from the consumption of A1 type milks.

Another priority should be to search for a human DNA based diagnostic assay which looks for the presence of the defect in the enzyme which in normal individuals should break down BCM-7. The enzyme is believed to be dipeptidyl-peptidase IV and is possibly absent or defective in autistics (and possibly schizophrenics and diabetics).

Under the NZDB funding NZDRI has performed work with the University of Auckland and thus far has also not been able to observe BCM-7 in the urine of limited number of normal people.

We have ethics approval to feed autistics A1 and A2 type milks and will examine their urine for the presence of BCM-7. This work will be performed early in 2001 and is NZDB funded.

We are also seeking ethics approval to perform a similar trial with diabetics. This work will be NZDB funded.

Trials are also planned to feed A1 and A2 to humans and look at factors that might be correlated with heart disease. In this way we hope to provide evidence that will prove or disprove A2 Corp. claims.

The NZ dairy industry has all of the capabilities needed for the production of A1 free milk. A limited amount of A2 milk could be produced relatively quickly using cow genotyping and the segregation of cows into specific herds.
Also attached is an earlier paper I prepared on the A1 and A2 situation which provides further details.

Jeremy Hill
8 October 2000

APPENDIX THREE

Lay summary provided by Professor Boyd Swinburn as part of his 2004 report to the NZ Food Safety Authority

Beta casein A1 and A2 in milk and human health: Lay Summary

About 25-30% of the protein in cows' milk is β-casein and it comes in several forms depending on the genetic make up of the cows. One of the forms is called A1 β-casein and it has been suggested that it might cause or aggravate one [sic] Type 1 diabetes (which is the type seen most commonly in children), heart disease, schizophrenia, and autism. The other main form of β-casein is called A2 and it has not been not been implicated in these diseases. The evidence to support the hypothesis that the A1/A2 composition of milk is a causative or protective factor in these diseases is reviewed in the report.

The strongest evidence is for Type 1 diabetes and heart disease. The main study supporting a relationship with the type of milk consumed was a comparison of 20 countries. Those countries with the highest consumption of A1 β-casein had the highest rates of Type 1 diabetes and heart disease. The relationship was very strong indeed, but these types of comparisons between countries can be difficult to interpret. There are many other factors that contribute to these diseases and the information is only averaged for the whole country's population. There have been a few other human and animal studies which provide some limited support for the hypothesis. Further research, especially involving human trials, is needed before it can be said with confidence that the A1/A2 composition of milk is important in human health.

The evidence in relation to an effect of A1 β-casein on schizophrenia or autism is much less. Some individuals with autism seem to improve on special diets that are free of both casein and gluten.

The A1/A2 hypothesis is both intriguing and potentially very important for population health if it is proved correct. It should be taken seriously and further research is needed. In addition, the appropriate government agencies have a responsibility to communicate the current state of evidence to the public, including the uncertainty about the evidence. Further public health actions, such as changing dietary advice or requiring labelling of milk products, are not considered to be warranted at this stage. Monitoring is also required to ensure that any claims made for A2 milk fall within the regulations for food claims.

Changing the dairy herds to more A2 producing cows is an option for the dairy and associated industries and these decisions will undoubtedly be made on a commercial basis. Changing dairy herds to more A2 producing cows may significantly improve public health, if the A1/A2 hypothesis is proved correct, and it is highly unlikely to do harm.

As a matter of individual choice, people may wish to reduce or remove A1 β-casein from their diet (or their children's diet) as a precautionary measure. This may be particularly relevant for those individuals who have or are at risk of the diseases mentioned (type 1 diabetes, coronary heart disease, autism and schizophrenia). However, they should do so knowing that there is substantial uncertainty about the benefits of such an approach.

INDEX

ABOUT THE AUTHOR

Keith Woodford is Professor of Farm Management and Agribusiness at Lincoln University in New Zealand. He is also a regular agribusiness commentator in the news media.

Keith has a Master of Agricultural Science from Lincoln University and a PhD from University of Queensland. For almost 20 years he lived in Australia, where he worked at University of Queensland, before returning to New Zealand in 2000. He has also worked on education, rural development and market research projects in more than 20 Asian and Pacific countries, funded by various development agencies such as NZAID, AusAID, UNDP, Asian Development Bank and Caritas Australia.

Keith is also a mountaineer. In his younger years he climbed in the Himalayas, Andes and Antarctica. At the time of the Erebus DC10 disaster in 1979 he was working in Antarctica as a survival instructor and was one of the first three people to land on the crash site, subsequently working alongside the accident investigators.

Keith lives in Christchurch with his family and remains committed to mountain-based activities.

the politics and practice of sustainable living

CHELSEA GREEN PUBLISHING

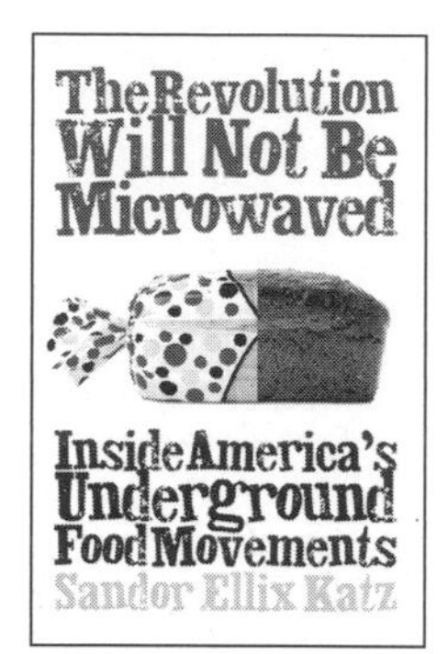

The Revolution Will Not Be Microwaved
Inside America's Underground
Food Movements
SANDOR ELLIX KATZ
ISBN 9781933392110
Paperback • $20

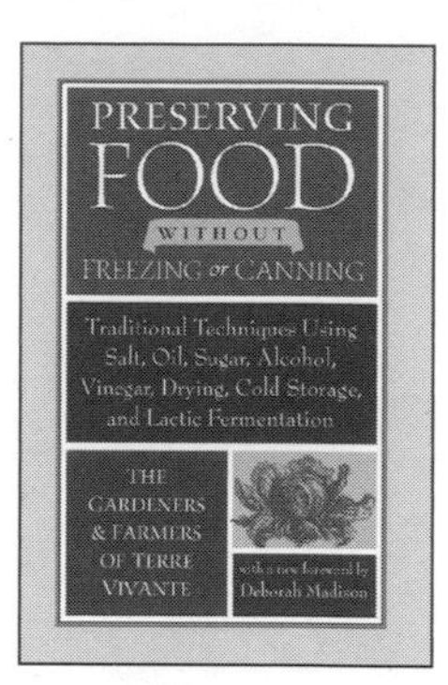

Preserving Food Without Freezing or Canning
Traditional Techniques Using Salt, Oil, Sugar, Alcohol,
Vinegar, Drying, Cold Storage, and Lactic Fermentation
THE GARDENERS & FARMERS OF TERRE VIVANTE
ISBN 9781933392592
Paperback • $25

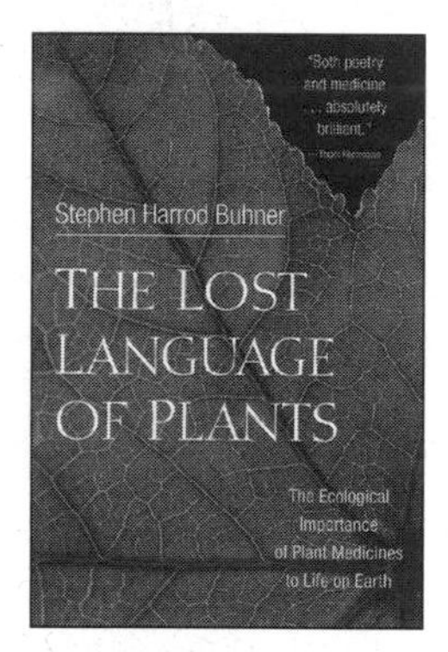

The Lost Language of Plants
The Ecological Importance of
Plant Medicines to Life on Earth
STEPHEN HARROD BUHNER
ISBN 9781890132880
Paperback • $19.95

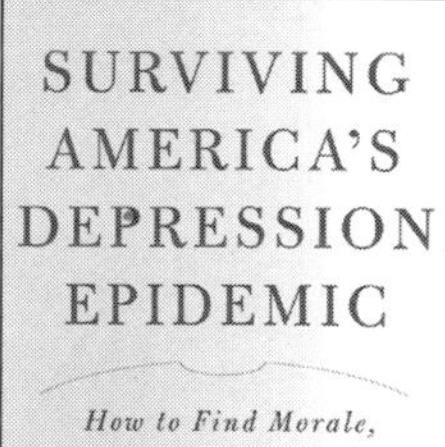

Surviving America's
Depression Epidemic
How to Find Morale, Energy, and
Community in a World Gone Crazy
BRUCE E. LEVINE, PhD
ISBN 9781933392714
Paperback • $16.95

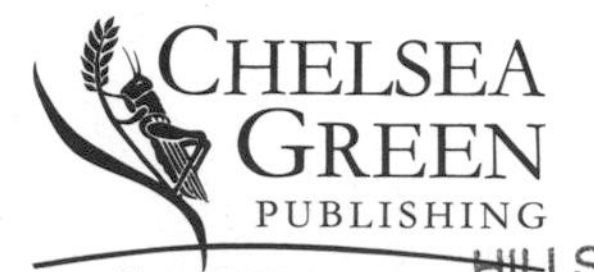

For more information or to request a catalog,
visit **www.chelseagreen.com** or
call toll-free **(800) 639-4099**.